FAST FACTS

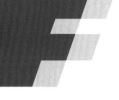

Epilepsy
Second edition

Indispensable

Guides to

Clinical

Practice

Martin J Brodie
Director, Epilepsy Unit,
Department of Medicine and Therapeutics,
Western Infirmary, Glasgow, UK

Steven C Schachter
Director, Clinical Research,
Comprehensive Epilepsy Center,
Beth Israel Deaconess Medical Center,
Boston, USA

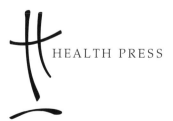

HEALTH PRESS

Oxford

Fast Facts – Epilepsy
First published 1999
Second edition 2001
Reprinted March 2004
Reprinted August 2005

Text © 2001 Martin J Brodie, Steven C Schachter
© 2001 in this edition Health Press Limited
Elizabeth House, Queen Street, Abingdon, Oxford OX14 3JR, UK

Tel: +44 (0)1235 523233
Fax: +44 (0)1235 523238

Fast Facts is a trade mark of Health Press Limited.

A CIP catalogue record for this title is available from the British Library.

ISBN 1-899541-69-1

Brodie, MJ (Martin)
Fast Facts – Epilepsy/
Martin J Brodie, Steven C Schachter

Printed by Fine Print (Services) Ltd, Oxford, UK.

Abbreviations

AED:	antiepileptic drug
CBZ:	carbamazepine
CLB:	clobazam
CNS:	central nervous system
CT:	computerized tomography
CZP:	clonazepam
EEG:	electroencephalogram
ESM:	ethosuximide
FBM:	felbamate
GBP:	gabapentin
JME:	juvenile myoclonic epilepsy
LEV:	levetiracetam
LTG:	lamotrigine
MRI:	magnetic resonance imaging
OXC:	oxcarbazepine
PB:	phenobarbital
PHT:	phenytoin
PRM:	primidone
SE:	status epilepticus
TGB:	tiagabine
TPM:	topiramate
VGB:	vigabatrin
VNS:	vagus nerve stimulation
VPA:	sodium valproate
ZNS:	zonisamide

Glossary

Cryptogenic seizures: partial-onset seizures with no identified underlying lesion

Cytochrome P450: a family of isoenzymes responsible for the hepatic oxidation of a range of lipid-soluble drugs

Enzyme inducer: a drug producing increased synthesis of hepatic drug metabolizing enzymes

Epilepsy: a tendency towards recurrent unprovoked seizures

Epilepsy syndrome: a constellation of characteristic seizures, abnormalities on EEG and/or brain imaging, prognosis with therapy, and associated clinical history and/or examination findings

Epileptogenesis: a sequence of events that converts a normal neuronal network into a hyperexcitable one

Generalized seizures: seizures initially involving both hemispheres usually with impairment of consciousness at the outset

Half-life: time taken for the plasma concentration of a drug to drop by 50%

Hypsarrhythmia: EEG pattern associated with infantile spasms, characterized by diffuse high voltage spike and slow waves, superimposed on a disorganized, slow background

Idiopathic seizures: seizures assumed to have a probable genetic basis

Incidence: the number of people developing epilepsy within a given time

Interictal: between epileptic seizures

Lennox-Gastaut: an encephalopathic syndrome of early childhood involving multiple seizure types, major abnormalities on the EEG, and usually mental retardation

Localization-related seizures: partial onset seizures arising from an identified lesion (also called symptomatic)

Partial seizure: a sudden, excessive, rapid and localized electrical discharge by grey matter from a particular part of the brain with or without impairment of consciousness

Pharmacogenomics: pharmacological targets identified from genetic mutations underlying epilepsy syndromes

Prevalence: the number of people with a diagnosis of epilepsy at any time

Pseudoseizure: a non-epileptic event feigning a seizure without any identifiable physiological abnormality

Seizure: the clinical manifestation of abnormal and excessive excitation of a population of cortical neurones

Steady state: the concentration achieved when the rate of drug administration equals the rate of drug elimination, occurring after around five elimination half-lives

Stevens-Johnson syndrome: severe idiosyncratic reaction characterized by skin eruption and mucosal and endothelial damage

West syndrome: the triad of infantile spasms, the typical EEG pattern of hypsarrhythmia, and arrest of psychomotor development

Introduction

Epilepsy is the most common serious neurological disorder in the world. Although this distressing condition remits in some people, many will have epilepsy throughout their lives. This dramatic disorder has had a place in the recorded history of all races and creeds since the dawn of literacy. Around 400 BC, Hippocrates considered epilepsy a sacred disease, but most cultures placed a demoniac interpretation on its unique constellation of symptoms and signs. It was only in 1875 that the English neurologist, John Hughlings Jackson, recognized a seizure as being due to disordered brain electricity.

There are a number of scientific and sociological revolutions surrounding the common and previously much-neglected subject of epilepsy. These have been fuelled by a better understanding of the pathophysiology of seizure propagation and generation, the appreciation of a widening range of seizure types and epilepsy syndromes, the development of more precise and accurate ways of imaging the brain, the introduction of a range of new antiepileptic drugs (AEDs) with different mechanisms of action, and the establishment of global patient advocacy organizations. In addition, epilepsy surgery has become more cost-effective than a lifetime of AED polypharmacy. These and other aspects of epilepsy will be discussed in this short, but practical, booklet designed to help the clinician diagnose and successfully treat patients with a wide range of seizure disorders.

Because of the rapid advances in our understanding of the treatment of epilepsy, this second edition has been published within 2 years of the first. Sections reflecting advances in the genetics of epilepsy and the treatment of special patient populations have been included, and two new AEDs have been added. We anticipate the need for regular updates to this slim volume during the coming decade.

CHAPTER 1
Epidemiology

Around 50 million people in the world have epilepsy. It is the commonest serious neurological condition with an annual incidence in developed countries of 50–70 cases per 100 000 of the population (Figure 1.1). In developing countries, the figure is higher due to more primitive obstetric services and the greater likelihood of cerebral infection and head trauma. The prevalence of epilepsy is around 1%. The incidence varies greatly with age, with high rates occurring in early childhood, falling to low levels in early adult life, but with a second peak in those aged over 65 years (Figure 1.2). In recent years, there has been a fall in the number of affected children accompanied by a sharp rise in epilepsy in the elderly. In many people, particularly children, the condition will remit, although a significant proportion will have epilepsy lifelong.

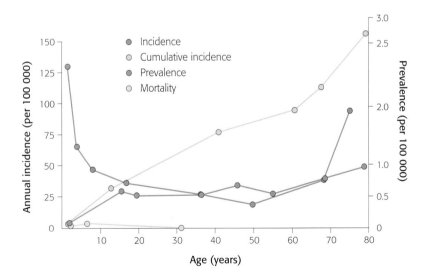

Figure 1.1 Incidence, prevalence and cumulative incidence rates for epilepsy in Rochester, Minnesota, 1940–1980. Reproduced with permission from Hauser *et al.* *Epilepsia* 1991;32:429–45.

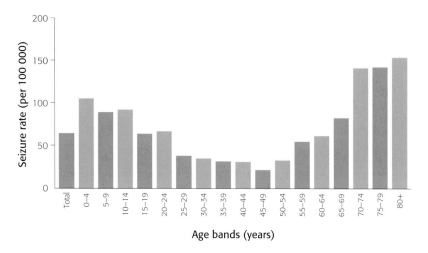

Figure 1.2 Incidence of epilepsy in relation to age. Reproduced with permission from Oxford University Press from Tallis *et al. Age Ageing* 1991;20:442–8.

The disease duration is often determined by the underlying cause. Sudden unexpected death, a complication of great concern, occurs in 1–5 per 1000 patient years, particularly if the seizure disorder remains uncontrolled.

CHAPTER 2
Diagnosis

Most specialists do not initiate pharmacological treatment routinely
following a single seizure, but will await a second or, occasionally, further
events if the situation remains unclear. A witness to one or more of the
episodes is an essential component to accurate diagnosis. A seizure is a
symptom and not a pathological process. It is, therefore, important to
determine whether the epilepsy is idiopathic and generalized (i.e. no seizure
warning or underlying brain lesion, often associated with a family history)
or symptomatic and localization-related (i.e. with aura, a specific site of
onset, an identifiable cause) by appropriate investigations, such as an
electroencephalogram (EEG) and brain imaging. Aetiology in relation to age
is shown in Figure 2.1. A number of factors can precipitate a seizure by
lowering the threshold in the brain for such an event (Table 2.1). For a
successful therapeutic outcome, the patient must understand the reason for
taking an AED and be convinced of the benefits of continuing treatment for

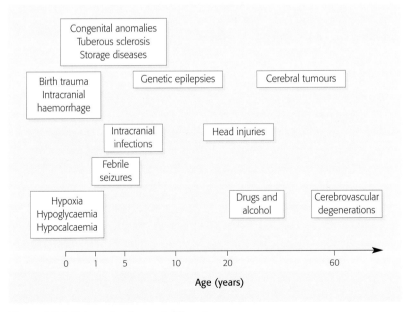

Figure 2.1 Aetiology of epilepsy at different ages.

11

TABLE 2.1

Factors lowering seizure threshold

Common	Occasional
• Sleep deprivation	• Dehydration
• Alcohol withdrawal	• Barbiturate withdrawal
• Television flicker	• Benzodiazepine withdrawal
• Epileptogenic drugs	• Hyperventilation
• Systemic infection	• Flashing lights
• Head trauma	• Diet and missed meals
• Recreational drugs	• Specific 'reflex' triggers
• AED non-compliance	• Stress
• Menstruation	• Intense exercise

some years. Accordingly, if there is doubt about the diagnosis despite a thorough evaluation or the patient's willingness to accept treatment after ample discussion, a wait-and-see policy is advised. Erratic compliance with medication, either as a consequence of lack of understanding of the prophylactic nature of the therapy or because of poor motivation, is a common reason for persisting seizures.

Seizure types

A seizure is a disturbance of movement, feeling or consciousness occasioned by sudden, inappropriate and excessive electrical discharges in the grey matter of the brain. Before initiating therapy, the clinician must establish the seizure type(s) by obtaining a thorough history from the patient and observers with particular attention to descriptions of actual seizures. This determination has important implications for the selection of AEDs, the likelihood of an underlying cerebral lesion, the prognosis and the possibility of genetic transmission. According to the classification established by the International League Against Epilepsy, seizures can be divided into two groups, partial and generalized (Table 2.2).

Partial seizures (Figure 2.2) originate in a focal region of the cortex and are subdivided into those that impair consciousness (complex partial) and those

TABLE 2.2

International classification of epileptic seizures

Partial seizures (beginning locally)

- Simple partial seizures (without impaired consciousness)
  - with motor symptoms
  - with somatosensory or special sensory symptoms
  - with autonomic symptoms
  - with psychological symptoms
- Complex partial seizures (with impaired consciousness)
  - simple partial onset followed by impaired consciousness
  - impaired consciousness at onset
- Partial seizures evolving into secondary generalized seizures

Generalized seizures (convulsive or non-convulsive)

- Absence seizures
  - typical
  - atypical
- Myoclonic seizures
- Clonic seizures
- Tonic seizures
- Tonic–clonic seizures
- Atonic seizures
- Unclassified seizures

that do not (simple partial). Both types of partial seizures can spread rapidly to other cortical areas through neuronal networks, resulting in secondary generalized tonic–clonic seizures (Figure 2.3). A simplified version of the seizure classification is shown in Table 2.3.

Simple partial seizures. The symptoms and signs of simple partial seizures depend on the site of origin of the abnormal electrical discharge. For example, those arising from the motor cortex cause rhythmic movements of the contralateral face, arm or leg (formerly called Jacksonian seizures). Seizures affecting sensory regions or those responsible for emotions

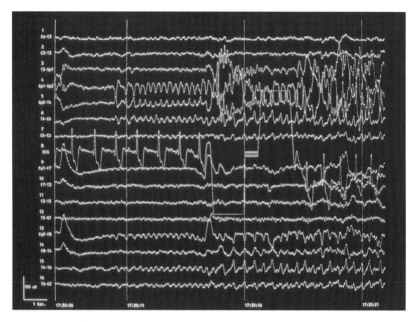

Figure 2.2 An EEG showing a focal seizure.

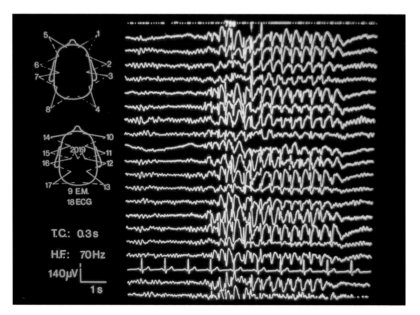

Figure 2.3 An EEG showing secondary generalization from a left frontal focus.

TABLE 2.3

Simplified classification of epileptic seizures

Partial seizures

- Simple – preservation of awareness
- Complex – impairment of consciousness
- Secondary generalized

Generalized seizures

- Absence
- Myoclonic
- Tonic–clonic
- Tonic
- Atonic

and memory may produce symptoms such as olfactory, visual or auditory hallucinations; *déjà vu* or *jamais vu*; and fear, panic or euphoria.

Complex partial seizures, previously called temporal lobe or psychomotor seizures, are the most common seizure type in adults and the most difficult to control with treatment. There may be a warning, called an aura (simple partial seizure), immediately preceding loss or reduction of awareness. Complex partial seizures typically last less than 3 minutes. During that time, patients may appear awake, but lose contact with their environment and do not respond normally to instructions or questions. Patients usually stare and either remain motionless or engage in repetitive semi-purposeful behaviour called automatisms, which may include the following: facial grimacing, gesturing, chewing, lip smacking, snapping fingers, repeating words or phrases, walking, running or even undressing. Patients are amnesic for these behaviours. If restrained during the seizure, they may become hostile or aggressive. After a seizure, patients are often sleepy and confused, and complain of a headache. This postictal state can vary from minutes to hours in duration.

Generalized seizures are characterized by widespread involvement of bilateral cortical regions at the outset, usually with impairment of consciousness. The familiar tonic–clonic seizure, often preceded by a cry, involves sudden falling to the ground followed by typical convulsive movements, sometimes with tongue or mouth biting and urinary incontinence. Other subtypes of generalized seizures include absence, myoclonic, clonic, tonic and atonic (see Table 2.3).

- Absence seizures mainly affect children, usually last 5–10 seconds, and commonly occur in clusters. They manifest as the sudden onset of staring with impaired consciousness with or without eye blinking and lip smacking. The EEG typically shows a 3 Hz spike and wave pattern (Figure 2.4). There is a strong genetic component for the seizures as well as for the EEG abnormality. While absences remit during adolescence in around 40% of patients, related tonic–clonic seizures may continue to occur into adulthood. Atypical absence seizures usually begin before 5 years of age and occur in conjunction with other generalized seizure types and mental retardation. They last longer than typical absence seizures and are often associated with changes in muscular tone.

- Myoclonic seizures consist of sudden, brief muscle contractions that may occur singly or in clusters, and can affect any group of muscles.

- Clonic seizures are characterized by rhythmic or semi-rhythmic muscle contractions, typically involving the upper extremities, neck and face.

- Tonic seizures cause sudden stiffening of extensor muscles, often associated with impaired consciousness and falling to the ground.

- Atonic seizures (drop attacks) produce the opposite effect, that is a sudden loss of muscle tone, with instantaneous collapse often resulting in facial or other injuries.

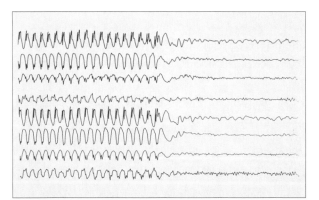

Figure 2.4 An EEG showing a 3 Hz spike and wave pattern reverting to normal.

Depression

Depression and suicide are four or five times more common in patients with epilepsy than in the general population. Ictal and postictal depressive symptoms may occur, but interictal depression is the most common presentation. Patients may not satisfy the diagnostic criteria of any of the DSM-IV affective disorders, but generally present with symptoms of depression with a chronic course interrupted by recurrent symptom-free periods of hours to several days.

Diagnosis is important because of the associated morbidity and mortality, but a high degree of suspicion is essential. Iatrogenic causes, particularly treatment with AEDs such as phenobarbital, primidone, vigabatrin and topiramate, must be excluded. Contributing psychosocial factors should be sought and addressed.

When choosing a suitable antidepressant, the selective serotonin re-uptake inhibitors are generally unlikely to exacerbate seizures. Monoamine oxidase inhibitors and non-tricyclic antidepressants are probably best avoided. Moclobemide and nefazodone may be exceptions as they do not appear to lower the seizure threshold.

CHAPTER 3
Epilepsy syndromes

In addition to the classification of seizures, there is a separate system for epilepsies and epileptic syndromes (Table 3.1). These are defined by groups of characteristic clinical features related to age of onset of seizures, family history of epilepsy, seizure type(s) and associated neurological symptoms and signs. Making a diagnosis of an epileptic syndrome allows the clinician to define the likely prognosis, provide reasonable genetic counselling and choose the most appropriate AED therapy. Epileptic syndromes are divided into those with generalized seizures (generalized epilepsies) and those with partial-onset seizures (localization-related or focal epilepsies). When the cause is known, it is called a symptomatic or secondary epilepsy; idiopathic (primary) or cryptogenic epilepsies have no identified cause. There are several epileptic syndromes that may be encountered by the family physician – benign rolandic epilepsy, juvenile myoclonic epilepsy, febrile convulsions, infantile spasms and Lennox-Gastaut syndrome.

Benign rolandic epilepsy

This is also called benign childhood epilepsy with centrotemporal spikes. It is an inherited disorder with onset from age 3 to 13 years that consists of predominantly nocturnal seizures and a characteristic pattern on the EEG. Affected patients have normal cognitive function and neurological examination. Seizures have a simple partial onset with occasional secondary generalization. Nocturnal seizures involve excessive salivation, gurgling or choking sounds, and clonic contractions of the mouth. Daytime seizures usually consist of tonic and/or clonic movements of one side of the body (particularly the face), speech arrest, and the preservation of consciousness. The EEG shows high-amplitude midtemporal-central spike and sharp waves, particularly during light sleep. The prognosis for children with benign rolandic epilepsy is excellent. These seizures are generally easy to control with AEDs and nearly all patients outgrow them.

Juvenile myoclonic epilepsy

Juvenile myoclonic epilepsy (JME) is an under-recognized syndrome characterized by myoclonic jerks, tonic–clonic seizures or clonic–tonic–clonic

TABLE 3.1

International classification of epilepsies and epileptic syndromes

Localization-related (focal, local or partial) epilepsies and syndromes

- Idiopathic epilepsy with age-related onset
  - benign childhood epilepsy with centrotemporal spikes
  - childhood epilepsy with occipital paroxysms
- Symptomatic epilepsy

Generalized epilepsies and syndromes

- Idiopathic epilepsy with age-related onset (listed in order of age at onset)
  - benign neonatal familial convulsions
  - benign neonatal non-familial convulsions
  - benign myoclonic epilepsy in infancy
  - childhood absence epilepsy (formerly known as pyknolepsy)
  - juvenile absence epilepsy
  - juvenile myoclonic epilepsy (formerly known as impulsive petit mal)
  - epilepsy with generalized tonic–clonic seizures on awakening
- Other idiopathic epilepsies
- Idiopathic or symptomatic epilepsy (listed in order of age at onset)
  - West syndrome (infantile spasms)
  - Lennox-Gastaut syndrome (childhood epileptic encephalopathy)
  - epilepsy with myoclonic–astatic seizures
  - epilepsy with myoclonic absence seizures
- Symptomatic epilepsy
- Non-specific syndromes
  - early myoclonic encephalopathy
  - early infantile epileptic encephalopathy
- Specific syndromes (epileptic seizures as a complication of a disease, such as phenylketonuria, juvenile Gaucher's disease or Lundborg's progressive myoclonic epilepsy)

TABLE 3.1 (continued)

Epilepsies and syndromes with both generalized and focal seizures

- Neonatal seizures
- Severe myoclonic epilepsy in infancy
- Epilepsy with continuous spike waves during slow-wave sleep
- Acquired epileptic aphasia (Landau–Kleffner syndrome)

Epilepsies without unequivocal generalized or focal features*

Special syndromes

- Situation-related seizures
  - febrile convulsions
  - seizures related to other identifiable situations, such as stress, hormonal changes, drugs, alcohol withdrawal or sleep deprivation
- Isolated, apparently unprovoked epileptic events
- Epilepsies characterized by specific modes of seizure precipitation
- Chronic progressive epilepsia partialis continua of childhood

*Includes cases in which the clinical and electroencephalographic findings do not permit classification of the epilepsy as clearly generalized or localization-related, such as cases of tonic–clonic seizures during sleep

seizures, and occasionally generalized absences (Figure 3.1). Myoclonic seizures occur within the first few hours after arising from sleep (as do the generalized seizures), are mild and bilaterally symmetrical, and usually involve the upper extremities without impairing consciousness. The patient may spill or drop things during a myoclonic jerk. Rarely, myoclonic seizures affecting the legs cause falls. JME is an inherited condition in otherwise neurologically normal children that usually begins during the teenage years. The seizures respond well to treatment, but usually relapse when medication is withdrawn. The EEG shows a characteristic 3.5–6 Hz spike-and-wave pattern and multiple spike-and-wave complexes that may be precipitated by photic stimulation and sleep deprivation.

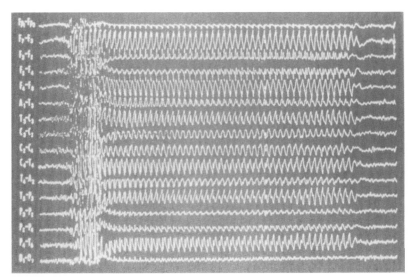

Figure 3.1 An EEG showing a myoclonic seizure followed by a generalized absence.

Febrile convulsions

These develop in association with fever (usually during the rapidly rising phase) without evidence of another defined cause. They typically present between the ages of 3 months and 5 years. The incidence is approximately 4% and there may be a family history of epilepsy. Up to 1 in 3 affected children will have recurrent febrile seizures. Febrile seizures are generally benign. Around 5% of children with febrile convulsions, however, later develop epilepsy.

Poor prognostic factors include seizures that have focal features or that last longer than 15 minutes, focal neurological abnormalities and a family history of afebrile seizures. Some of these children will go on to develop mesial temporal sclerosis and partial seizures that are often refractory to AED therapy. Treatment of febrile convulsions is usually symptomatic with prompt administration of an antipyretic and sponge bathing. Some physicians advocate prophylactic rectal diazepam when fever occurs in children with a previous history of febrile convulsions. Most paediatric neurologists would not recommend long-term AED treatment for children with simple febrile seizures (i.e. generalized seizures lasting < 15 minutes).

21

Infantile spasms

Infantile spasms are sudden, brief seizures that are typically tonic flexor spasms of the waist, extremities and neck. They are usually seen as part of West's syndrome, which is defined as infantile spasms, hypsarrhythmic patterns on the EEG, and severe encephalopathy with psychomotor retardation. The mortality rate is 20% and death usually results from the underlying pathology. Among infants who survive, over 75% are mentally retarded and over 50% continue to have seizures throughout life. The aetiology may be known, such as cerebral malformations (half of all patients with tuberous sclerosis develop infantile spasms), perinatal brain damage, and postnatal cerebral insults, or it may be idiopathic. Spasms typically begin before the age of 1 year, with a peak occurrence of onset between 4 and 6 months of age. Seizures may occur dozens, if not hundreds, of times daily. In addition to massive flexor spasms, abduction or adduction of the arms, self-hugging movements and extensor contractions of the neck and trunk may be seen. The EEG is markedly abnormal in the majority of cases and consists of diffuse high-voltage spike and slow waves superimposed on a disorganized, slow background (hypsarrhythmia).

Lennox-Gastaut syndrome

Lennox-Gastaut syndrome is a devastating disorder in children that consists of mixed types of seizures, slow (< 2.5 Hz) spike-and-wave EEG patterns superimposed on an abnormal, slow background, and progressive mental retardation. Seizures typically occur daily, often in the tens or hundreds, and consist of axial tonic, tonic–clonic, atypical absence, myoclonic and atonic seizures, which often cause injuries. The tonic seizures usually occur during the night, sometimes in clusters, and are brief. Atonic seizures may vary from head drops to catastrophic falls. Cognitive deficit is usually present before the seizures develop and may be associated with behavioural problems. Most children demonstrate abnormalities on neurological examination. Prognosis for seizure remission is poor and response to AED therapy is generally unsatisfactory.

Genetics

Genetics has been one of the more exciting areas of progress in the field of epilepsy in recent years. A number of hereditary epilepsies have been linked to genes that encode ion channels or functionally related proteins. Specifically, three forms of autosomal dominant inherited human epilepsy have been identified. Benign familial neonatal convulsions, which begin in the first few days of life and usually disappear by the sixth week, occur in otherwise phenotypically normal infants. Linkage studies have tied this disorder to mutations of voltage-gated potassium channels. Generalized epilepsy with febrile seizures plus is characterized by a history of febrile seizures that may have delayed resolution. In addition, family members may have other seizure types, usually associated with primary generalized epilepsy. In one Australian family, this disorder has been mapped to chromosome 19q, which encodes a voltage-sensitive sodium channel subunit.

A partial epilepsy syndrome, previously found to have autosomal dominant transmission, has now been associated with a mutation in a central nicotinic acetylcholine receptor. This disorder, autosomal dominant nocturnal frontal lobe epilepsy, does not develop until later in childhood and may persist into adulthood. Phenotypically and electrographically, it is similar to acquired frontal lobe epilepsies. However, neuroimaging is unremarkable and the disorder responds readily to AED therapy. Identifying the channel abnormalities that lead to an expression of epilepsy will potentially provide an insight into the mechanisms of excitability and seizure production, not only in genetically predetermined epilepsy but also in acquired types. Pharmacogenomics will provide a range of novel targets for AED development.

CHAPTER 4
Diagnostic techniques

Electroencephalography

Electroencephalography is useful to confirm the clinical diagnosis of epilepsy and to support the classification of partial-onset or generalized seizures. Standard EEGs are insensitive in that more than 50% of patients with epilepsy will have a normal routine trace. Activation techniques, including hyperventilation and photic stimulation (Figure 4.1), can be helpful in uncovering abnormalities. If the initial EEG is unremarkable and the diagnosis is in doubt, a sleep-deprivation study is recommended. Providing the electroencephalographer with detailed information concerning the patient's age, seizure behaviour and response to AEDs is important. EEGs have a limited role in determining whether a patient may have their seizure medication safely tapered after a prolonged seizure-free interval. In a patient suspected to have non-convulsive status epilepticus, an EEG

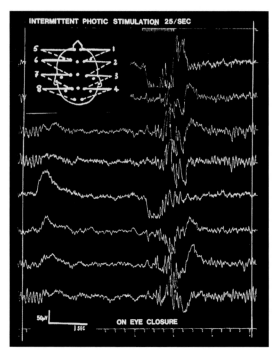

Figure 4.1

Photoconvulsive response provoked by intermittent photic stimulation.

may be diagnostic and can immediately differentiate between convulsive status and pseudostatus epilepticus.

Brain imaging

Imaging studies of the brain are essential to the appropriate evaluation of most patients with epilepsy, particularly those presenting with partial-onset seizures. Computerized tomography (CT) and magnetic resonance imaging (MRI) allow identification of structural lesions, but MRI has higher sensitivity and specificity, particularly for localizing developmental disorders (Figure 4.2), cortical dysgenesis (Figure 4.3), hippocampal sclerosis, arteriovenous malformations and gliomas (Figure 4.4). CT scanning should be performed if MRI is unavailable, or in patients for whom MRI is contraindicated (e.g. those with pacemakers, non-compatible aneurysm clips, severe claustrophobia).

Structural lesions that underlie seizures are found in up to 50% of cases; typical pathological findings vary with age. Among children, an MRI is particularly useful in identifying congenital abnormalities, such as neuronal migration disorders and arteriovenous malformations. In young adulthood, frequently detected conditions are mesial temporal sclerosis, sequelae of head trauma, congenital anomalies, brain tumours and vascular lesions. In mid-life and beyond, scans will be helpful in evaluating stroke and cerebral degeneration, and in identifying primary and secondary neoplasia.

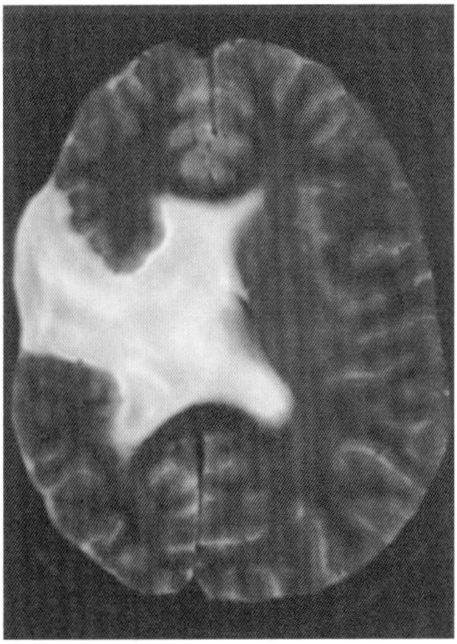

Patients with partial-onset seizures or epileptic syndromes known to be associated with brain structural pathology should undergo an MRI procedure as part of their initial diagnostic evaluation. Patients with refractory epilepsy whose initial MRI is normal should have a high-resolution study to exclude hippocampal atrophy and focal cortical dysplasia.

Figure 4.2 MRI showing schizencephaly.

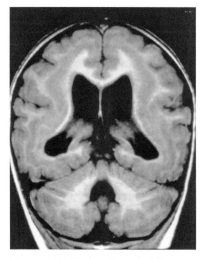 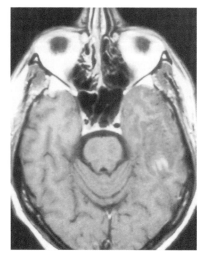

Figure 4.3 MRI showing a double cortex.

Figure 4.4 MRI showing right-sided grade III glioma.

The scan should be repeated periodically if there is one of the following:

- suspicion of a tumour
- worsening in the patient's neurological examination or cognitive function
- deterioration in the frequency or severity of the seizures.

Other neuroimaging techniques, such as single-photon emission CT, positron emission tomography, MR spectroscopy and functional MRI, may identify functional cerebral changes underlying structural abnormalities and are useful adjuncts in patients being considered for epilepsy surgery. These investigations have a limited role in routine diagnostic evaluation.

CHAPTER 5

Pharmacological treatment

Starting treatment

Most patients reporting more than one well-documented or witnessed seizure require treatment. Exceptions can include widely separated seizures, provoked seizures for which avoidance activity may be sufficient prophylaxis (e.g. concomitant illness, photosensitive epilepsy, alcohol withdrawal) and patients unlikely or unwilling to take medication (e.g. alcohol abusers, drug addicts, conscientious objectors). The information should be presented to the patient in the context of what is known and what is conjecture about the risk of recurrent seizures, the chance of a successful outcome with treatment, and the likelihood of remission. In this way, the patient can make an informed commitment to the treatment plan. More controversial is the issue of whether to treat a single seizure. Patients who experience an unprovoked seizure have a significant chance of recurrence over the next 5 years, varying from 31 to 71% depending on the study. Those with an underlying cerebral lesion and an abnormal EEG or who have a high-risk epilepsy syndrome, such as JME, have the greatest likelihood of recurrence and probably should be treated after their first seizure. In a few specific epilepsy syndromes, such as simple febrile seizures and benign rolandic epilepsy, pharmacotherapy may be unnecessary.

The decision whether or not to start treatment should be made after ample discussion with the patient and his or her family of the risks and benefits of both courses of action. Never push the issue if there is doubt about the diagnosis, particularly if the patient resists the introduction of AED therapy. The goal should be maintenance of a normal lifestyle by complete seizure control without side-effects. When prescribing an AED, the clinician *must* discuss all common side-effects, including the risk of teratogenesis in women of child-bearing potential. That the latter has been touched upon should be documented in the patient's case notes. Similarly, regulations regarding driving should be raised and documented. Time should be taken to deal with the patient's fears, misconceptions and prejudices, as

27

TABLE 5.1

Pharmacokinetics of established antiepileptic drugs

Drug	Absorption (bioavailability %)	Protein binding (% bound)
Carbamazepine	Slow (75–80)	70–80
Clobazam	Rapid (90–100)	87–90
Clonazepam	Rapid (80–90)	80–90
Ethosuximide	Rapid (90–95)	0
Phenobarbital	Slow (95–100)	48–54
Phenytoin	Slow (85–90)	90–93
Primidone	Rapid (90–100)	20–30
Sodium valproate	Rapid (100)	88–92

well as those of the family. The importance of total compliance with medication should also be stressed. These issues often require amplification at subsequent visits.

A single drug (monotherapy) should be introduced at low doses with increments over a number of weeks (depending on the AED and the urgency of the situation) to establish an effective and tolerable regimen. This will help avoid concentration-dependent side-effects, in particular central nervous system (CNS) toxicity, the presence of which is likely to discourage the patient from persevering with therapy long term. An additional benefit of a cautious approach is that it allows tolerance to develop to sedation or cognitive impairment. Such a policy will also detect early the emergence of potentially serious idiosyncratic reactions, such as rash, hepatotoxicity and blood dyscrasias. Measuring the serum drug

Elimination half-life (hours)	Routes of elimination	Target range
24–45 (single) 8–24 (chronic)	• Hepatic metabolism • Active metabolite	4–12 mg/litre (17–50 µmol/litre)
10–30	• Hepatic metabolism • Active metabolite	None
30–40	• Hepatic metabolism	None
20–60	• Hepatic metabolism • 25% excreted unchanged	40–100 mg/litre (283–706 µmol/litre)
72–144	• Hepatic metabolism • 25% excreted unchanged	10–40 mg/litre (40–172 µmol/litre)
9–40	• Saturable hepatic metabolism	10–20 mg/litre (40–80 µmol/litre)
4–12	• Hepatic metabolism • Active metabolites • 40% excreted unchanged	8–12 mg/litre (25–50 µmol/litre)
7–17	• Hepatic metabolism • Active metabolites	50–100 mg/litre (350–700 µmol/litre)

concentration when steady state has been reached will confirm appropriate compliance, and provide a useful baseline for further dosing if seizure control is not complete.

Established antiepileptic drugs

Despite the recent entry into the market place of a range of new pharmacological treatments, most patients still receive treatment with the established AEDs. Comparative pharmacokinetics, indications and a guide to dosing in children and adults are summarized in Tables 5.1, 5.2 and 5.3. Their efficacies against common seizure types and syndromes are illustrated in Table 5.4. The use of each drug will be considered, highlighting the problems likely to be encountered in everyday clinical practice.

TABLE 5.2

Dosing guidelines for established antiepileptic drugs in adults

Drug	Indications	Starting daily dose (mg)
Carbamazepine	• Partial and tonic–clonic seizures	200
Clobazam	• Partial and generalized seizures	10
Clonazepam	• Myoclonic and tonic–clonic seizures • Status epilepticus	1
Ethosuximide	• Absence seizures	500
Phenobarbital	• Partial and tonic–clonic, myoclonic, clonic and tonic seizures • Status epilepticus	60
Phenytoin	• Partial and tonic–clonic seizures • Status epilepticus	200
Primidone	• Partial and tonic–clonic seizures	125
Sodium valproate	• All generalized seizures • Partial seizures	500

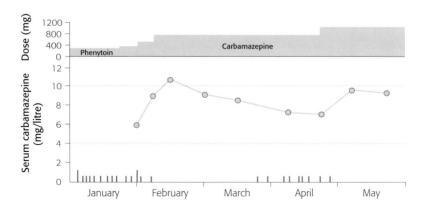

Figure 5.1 Auto-induction of carbamazepine metabolism. The lines at the bottom of the graph represent partial (short) and tonic–clonic (longer) seizures.

Commonest daily dose (mg)	Maintenance daily dose (mg)	Dosage interval*
600	400–2000	bd–qds
20	10–40	od–bd
4	2–8	od–bd
1000	500–2000	od–bd
120	60–240	od–bd
300	100–700	od–bd
500	250–1500	od–bd
1000	500–3000	bd–tds

*od, once daily; bd, twice daily; tds, three times a day; qds, four times a day

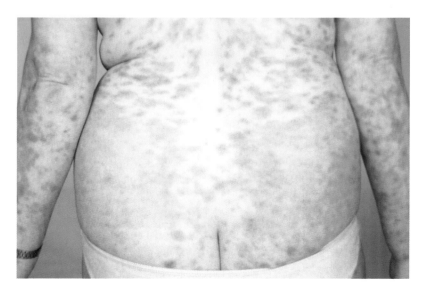

Figure 5.2 Typical morbilliform rash due to carbamazepine.

31

TABLE 5.3

Dosing guidelines for established antiepileptic drugs in children

Drug	Starting dose	Maintenance dose (mg/kg/day)	Dosage interval* (mg/kg/day)
Carbamazepine	5	10–25	bd–qds
Clobazam	0.25	0.5–1	od–bd
Clonazepam	0.025	0.025–0.1	bd–tds
Ethosuximide	10	15–30	od–bd
Phenobarbital	4	4–8	od–bd
Phenytoin	5	5–15	od–bd
Primidone	10	20–30	od–bd
Sodium valproate	10	15–40	bd–tds

*od, once daily; bd, twice daily; tds, three times a day; qds, four times a day

TABLE 5.4

Efficacy of established antiepileptic drugs against common seizure types and syndromes

Drug	Partial	Secondary generalized	Tonic–clonic	Absence	Myoclonic	Lennox-Gastaut	Infantile spasms
Carbamazepine	+	+	+	–	–	0	0
Clobazam	+	+	+	?	+	+	?+
Clonazepam	+	+	+	?	+	?+	?+
Ethosuximide	0	0	0	+	0	0	0
Phenobarbital	+	+	+	0	?+	?	?
Phenytoin	+	+	+	–	–	0	0
Primidone	+	+	+	0	?	?	?
Sodium valproate	+	+	+	+	+	+	+

+, proven efficacy; ?+, probable efficacy; 0, ineffective; –, worsens control; ?, unknown

Carbamazepine (CBZ) was synthesized by Schindler at Geigy in 1953 in an attempt to compete with the newly introduced antipsychotic chlorpromazine. The first clinical studies in epilepsy were not carried out until 1963. Over the years, CBZ has slowly gained acceptance as a first-line treatment for partial and tonic–clonic seizures. It is not effective, and may even be deleterious, for generalized absences and myoclonic seizures. CBZ acts by preventing repetitive firing of action potentials in depolarized neurones via use- and voltage-dependent blockade of sodium channels.

CBZ should be introduced in low doses (100–200 mg daily) with 100–200 mg increments every 3–14 days, depending on the urgency of the situation. Slow introduction will facilitate tolerance to its CNS side-effects and allow hepatic auto-induction of CBZ metabolism to take place. The dose can be increased over the first month or two to a maintenance dose that completely controls the seizure disorder. A balance must be achieved in the individual patient between speed of seizure control and acceptance of temporary CNS toxicity. The final dose will depend on the extent to which CBZ induces its own metabolism (Figure 5.1). Despite this careful approach, some patients will be unable to tolerate the neurotoxic side-effects of CBZ, even at low doses and serum concentrations. Diplopia, headache, dizziness, nausea and vomiting are the commonest complaints. For many patients with refractory epilepsy, these symptoms provide a dose ceiling, which may be less than an effective dose. High peak concentrations often result in intermittent side-effects around 2 hours after dosing, necessitating three or four times daily administration in some patients. Such problems can be overcome by prescribing a controlled-release formulation that can be given twice daily, or by shifting a greater percentage of the total daily dose to bedtime, particularly when the patient has only nocturnal or early morning seizures.

CBZ can cause a range of idiosyncratic reactions, the most common of which is a morbilliform rash in around 10% of patients (Figure 5.2). Other unusual, but more severe, skin eruptions include erythema multiforme and Stevens-Johnson syndrome. Reversible mild leucopenia often occurs within the first few months of treatment, but does not require discontinuation of therapy unless accompanied by evidence of infection or if the white cell count slips well below 2000 x 10^9/litre. Potentially fatal blood dyscrasias and toxic hepatitis are much rarer problems. At high concentrations, the drug has an antidiuretic hormone-like action that can result in fluid retention in patients with cardiac failure and in the elderly. Mild hyponatraemia is usually asymptomatic, but if the serum sodium falls below 120 mmol/litre, the patient may present with confusion, peripheral oedema and a deterioration in seizure control. CBZ is teratogenic and, in particular, is associated with an incidence of around 0.5% of spina bifida in exposed fetuses.

As well as inducing its own metabolism, CBZ can accelerate the hepatic breakdown of a number of lipid-soluble drugs. The most common interaction is with the oral contraceptive pill, necessitating a daily oestrogen dose of 50 µg or more for most women. Other important targets include sodium valproate (VPA), ethosuximide (ESM), corticosteroids, anticoagulants, antipsychotics and cyclosporin. Drugs that inhibit CBZ metabolism resulting in toxicity include phenytoin (PHT), cimetidine, danazol, dextropropoxyphene, diltiazem, erythromycin, isoniazid, verapamil, viloxazine and fluoxetine. The substantial variation in any given patient in CBZ concentrations over the course of a day – as much as 100% with twice-daily dosing – makes the interpretation of concentration monitoring problematical unless the times of dosing and blood sampling are standardized. In many patients, the dose can be titrated adequately on clinical criteria alone. Exceptions include those in whom compliance is suspect and those taking a cocktail of AEDs likely to interact with one another.

Phenytoin. The discovery and clinical testing of PHT by Merritt and Putnam in the 1930s introduced both a major new non-sedating AED and an animal model of epilepsy (electrical seizures in the cat). For the past 60 years, PHT has been a first-line medication for the prevention of partial and tonic–clonic seizures and for the acute treatment of seizures and status epilepticus. PHT is not effective against myoclonic, atonic and absence seizures. It is available in oral and intravenous forms; a recently introduced prodrug, fosphenytoin, can be given intravenously or intramuscularly when urgent intervention is indicated. Like CBZ, PHT blocks voltage-dependent neuronal sodium channels.

Depending on the urgency of the situation, PHT may be started at the maintenance dose, typically 300 mg/day in two divided doses in adults (5–8 mg/kg/day in children), or more rapidly (e.g. 20 mg/kg divided into three oral doses over 24 hours, or 20 mg/kg given intravenously – no faster than 50 mg/minute for parenteral PHT or 150 mg/minute for fosphenytoin). The dose should be increased at 1–2 weekly increments as necessary and as tolerated. Most adults usually achieve satisfactory seizure control with once-daily dosing. Patients with erratic compliance should be treated twice daily to lessen the effect of a missed dose.

PHT is metabolized in the liver; the first step of this process involves the enzyme arene oxidase, which has saturable kinetics, particularly at moderate-to-high serum concentrations. The concentration at which PHT pharmacokinetics become non-linear varies as a function of age. As a consequence of this pharmacokinetic profile, small changes in dosing may result in disproportionate changes in serum concentration (Figure 5.3). In all patients, the dose should be increased or decreased by 25–50 mg increments when clinically indicated, particularly when serum concentrations exceed 10 mg/litre. Serum concentrations should then be checked 1–2 weeks later. Side-effects of PHT can be divided into neurotoxic symptoms (ataxia, nystagmus, dysarthria, asterixis, somnolence) that typically present 8–12 hours after an oral dose, chronic dysmorphic effects (gingival hyperplasia, hirsutism, acne, facial coarsening) that occur after months of therapy, and long-term problems (folate deficiency, osteopenia, peripheral neuropathy, cerebellar atrophy) that are uncommon and take years to develop. PHT is associated with rash in approximately 5% of patients.

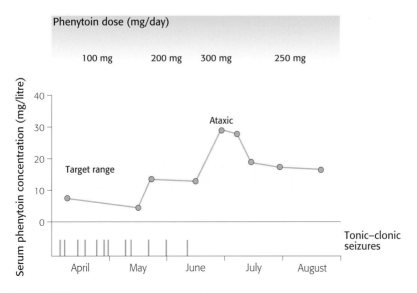

Figure 5.3 Saturation kinetics with phenytoin.

Other rare idiosyncratic reactions include Stevens-Johnson syndrome, hepatitis, bone marrow suppression, lymphadenopathy and a lupus-like syndrome. PHT is also a weak teratogen.

PHT produces hepatic enzyme induction and may, therefore, reduce serum concentrations of metabolized AEDs such as CBZ, VPA and primidone (PRM). The effectiveness of other lipid-soluble drugs including oral contraceptives and anticoagulants is also jeopardized. PHT is tightly bound to circulating albumin and may be displaced by other drugs, some of which, like VPA, also inhibit its metabolism. Checking free PHT serum concentrations may be useful clinically to correlate with a patient's possible neurotoxic symptoms in the setting of hypoalbuminaemia, renal and hepatic insufficiency, or pregnancy. Febrile illness may increase the clearance of PHT, resulting in lowered serum concentrations. Enteral feeding has been reported to decrease PHT absorption.

Sodium valproate. VPA's anticonvulsant property was recognized serendipitously in 1963, when it was used by Pierre Eymard as a solvent for a number of other compounds. It is now established as effective over the complete range of seizure types, with particular value for the idiopathic generalized epilepsies. VPA exerts its antiepileptic property, at least in part, by limiting sustained repetitive firing by a use- and voltage-dependent effect on sodium channels. It also facilitates the effects of the inhibitory neurotransmitter, γ-aminobutyric acid (GABA).

The starting dose for adults and adolescents should be 500 mg once or twice daily. Alterations thereafter can be made according to the clinical status of the patient. Divalproex sodium (a combination of valproic acid and VPA) can also be given twice daily. As the drug can take several weeks to become fully effective, frequent dose adjustments shortly after initiating therapy may be unwarranted. Because VPA does not exhibit a clear-cut concentration–effect–toxicity relationship and daily variations in concentration at a given dose are wide, routine monitoring is not helpful unless closely correlated with the patient's clinical situation. A few patients need and tolerate serum concentrations up to 150 mg/litre.

Unpleasant side-effects with VPA include dose-related tremor, weight gain due to appetite stimulation, thinning or loss of hair (usually temporary), and menstrual irregularities including amenorrhoea. Some young women develop polycystic ovarian syndrome associated with obesity and hirsutism. Rarely, stupor and encephalopathy can occur. Sedation is an uncommon complaint. Hepatotoxicity, histologically a microvesicular steatosis similar to that found in Reye's syndrome, affects fewer than 1 in 20 000 exposed individuals. This appears to be a particular concern in children under 3 years of age receiving AED polypharmacy, some of whom will have a coexistent metabolic defect. Other sporadic problems include thrombocytopenia and pancreatitis. VPA can inhibit a range of hepatic metabolic processes, including oxidation, conjugation and epoxidation reactions. Targets include other AEDs, particularly PHT, phenobarbital (PB), the active epoxide metabolite of CBZ and lamotrigine. VPA does not, however, interfere metabolically with the hormonal components of the oral contraceptive pill.

Ethosuximide. Since its introduction in 1958, ESM has been the drug of choice for children with absence seizures who do not also have tonic–clonic or myoclonic seizures. ESM is also effective for atypical absences, but ineffective for myoclonic, tonic–clonic and partial-onset seizures. It works by reducing T-type calcium currents in thalamic neurones. The metabolism of ESM is hepatic, protein binding is minimal, and drug interactions are not a major problem. Side-effects occur in approximately 40% of patients and predominantly relate to the gastrointestinal tract (hiccups, nausea, vomiting, abdominal pain, anorexia). Headache, dizziness, drowsiness and unsteadiness may also occur. Allergic rashes are seen in up to 5% of patients. A transient leucopenia has been described. In adults, dosing is initiated with 500 mg daily (250 mg/day in children < 6 years old) with 250 mg dose increments as clinically indicated over 2–3 weeks to the maximum tolerated amount, which is typically 15–40 mg/kg given two or three times daily. Serum concentrations less than 40 mg/litre are usually ineffective.

Phenobarbital is the oldest AED in common clinical use. Once widely prescribed for partial and tonic–clonic seizures, it is now generally regarded as second-line therapy because it so often causes sedation and behavioural problems, such as depression and agitation. Hyperactivity may occur in children and elderly patients. The parenteral formulation of PB is occasionally useful as adjunctive therapy in status epilepticus. PB may also be used for myoclonic seizures. It enhances the effect of GABA by prolonging chloride channel opening at the $GABA_A$ receptor resulting in neuronal hyperpolarization.

PB is metabolized in the liver, and is a powerful inducer of hepatic metabolism, accelerating the clearance of many other lipid-soluble drugs. The half-life of PB is 4 days. Consequently, steady-state serum concentrations may not be reached for up to 3 weeks after a change in dose. In children, doses of 2–5 mg/kg daily are usually necessary for optimal seizure control. Resulting serum concentrations typically range from 15 to 40 mg/litre. Tapering PB medication should be attempted very slowly (e.g. 15 mg/month) to minimize the possibility of withdrawal seizures and other unpleasant symptoms, such as altered mood and sleep disturbance.

Primidone. PRM is metabolized in the liver to PB and another active substance, phenylethylmalonamide. PRM is as effective as CBZ, PHT and PB for partial-onset seizures, but has a higher incidence of side-effects, particularly sedation and ataxia. Because of its relative poor tolerability, it is primarily used as adjunctive therapy. As its half-life is shorter than that of PB, concentrations of PB are usually higher than those of PRM. Dosing should be started with 125 mg at bedtime, increasing by 125 mg every 3–5 days as tolerated to 500–1500 mg daily in two or three divided doses. As with PB, discontinuation of PRM should be undertaken very gradually.

Clonazepam. Like other benzodiazepines, clonazepam (CZP) enhances GABA-mediated inhibition and is primarily used as adjunctive treatment for myoclonic and atonic seizures. Parenteral CZP can be used for status epilepticus. Drug interactions are minimal and the half-life is approximately 24 hours. Side-effects are prominent, usually dose-limiting, and include sedation, ataxia and behavioural changes, such as depression. Adults should be started on 0.5–1.0 mg/day with subsequent weekly increments as necessary. In children, 0.5 mg per day is the usual starting dose. Tolerance to the anticonvulsant effect and difficulty weaning patients off CZP limit its clinical value.

Clobazam (CLB) is a useful adjunctive drug in refractory epilepsy. Not all responders will maintain a worthwhile improvement in seizure control on long-term dosing due to the development of tolerance. Some of these will have an anatomical basis for their seizure disorder. Nevertheless, a significant proportion (10–20%) of patients treated with CLB become seizure-free. Intermittent use of CLB reduces the likelihood of tolerance. Short-term administration (e.g. 20 mg daily for 3 days) can be an effective strategy in women with premenstrual seizure exacerbations and as 'cover' for holidays or stressful events, such as weddings and surgery. A single dose of 30 mg can have a useful prophylactic action if taken immediately after the first event in patients who suffer regular clusters of complex partial and secondary generalized seizures. CLB's structure (1,5-benzodiazepine) differs slightly from those of clonazepam and diazepam (1,4-benzodiazepines), and this may account for a lower propensity to produce sedation. Nevertheless, depression, irritability and tiredness are reported. As with barbiturates, deterioration in behaviour and mood disturbance can occur, particularly in patients with learning disabilities in whom CLB should probably be avoided. CLB is not available in the USA.

Newer antiepileptic drugs

During the 1990s, after a hiatus of nearly 20 years, nine new AEDs (and one device – the vagus nerve stimulator) have received licences for the adjunctive treatment of refractory epilepsy. Some of these can also be used as monotherapy in less severe seizure disorders. Lamotrigine (LTG), gabapentin (GBP), vigabatrin (VGB) and oxcarbazepine (OXC) are widely available, though VGB is not licensed in the USA. Topiramate (TPM), tiagabine (TGB), levetiracetam (LEV) and zonisamide (ZNS) are in the process of being marketed around the world. The progress of felbamate (FBM) has been dramatically curtailed because of the unusual development of idiosyncratic life-threatening bone-marrow and liver toxicity. The advent of these newer treatments has provided many more options in the management of refractory epilepsy, and some of these, particularly LTG, GBP and OXC have the potential to become first-line drugs as monotherapy in newly diagnosed epilepsy. Their kinetics, dosing in adults and children, and range of efficacy are highlighted in Tables 5.5, 5.6, 5.7 and 5.8, respectively.

Lamotrigine is licensed widely as add-on treatment for adults with refractory epilepsy. Its use in children and as monotherapy in newly diagnosed epilepsy

TABLE 5.5

Pharmacokinetics of new antiepileptic drugs

Drug	Absorption (bioavailability %)	Protein binding (%)	Half-life* (hours)	Route(s) of elimination
Felbamate	Slow (95–100)	22–36	13–23	• Hepatic metabolism • Renal excretion
Gabapentin	Slow (60)	0	5–7	• Renal excretion
Lamotrigine	Rapid (95–100)	55	22–36	• Metabolized to glucuronide conjugate
Levetiracetam	Rapid (95–100)	< 10	7–8	• Renal excretion
Oxcarbazepine	Rapid (95–100)	40†	8–10†	• Hepatic conversion to active moiety
Tiagabine	Rapid (95–100)	96	5–9	• Hepatic metabolism
Topiramate	Slow (80)	9–17	20–24	• Renal excretion • Hepatic metabolism
Vigabatrin	Slow (60–80)	0	5–7	• Renal excretion
Zonisamide	Rapid (95–100)	40–60	50–68	• Hepatic meabolism • Renal excretion

*As monotherapy
†Parameters for active metabolite, 10-OH-carbazepine

has been approved in a growing number of countries. It selectively blocks the slow inactivated state of the sodium channel, thereby preventing the release of excitatory amino-acid neurotransmitters, particularly glutamate and aspartate. This effect does not explain its anti-absence and anti-myoclonic properties. LTG appears to be effective across the complete range of seizure types, including partial seizures, the idiopathic generalized epilepsies and Lennox-Gastaut syndrome. Good results have been reported in patients with learning disabilities who often have multiple seizure types. LTG's ability to reduce interictal spiking may explain the improved alertness reported by some patients taking the drug. Its efficacy may be enhanced when combined with VPA, although this combination is associated with higher rates of rash and tremor.

The commonest side-effects with LTG are headache, nausea, insomnia, vomiting, dizziness, diplopia, ataxia and tremor. Sedation seldom occurs with the drug. Rash complicates initial management in around 5% of patients. It is usually maculopapular and, in mild cases, may subside spontaneously without drug withdrawal. In a few patients, however, there is an accompanying systemic illness with malaise, fever, arthralgia, myalgia, lymphadenopathy and eosinophilia. Cases of bullous erythema multiforme, Stevens-Johnson syndrome and toxic epidermal necrolysis have also been reported. The risk of a severe skin reaction may be as high as 1:1000 and 1:100 in adults and children, respectively. Gradual introduction of LTG lessens the incidence of rash, the development of

TABLE 5.6

Dosing guidelines for new antiepileptic drugs in adults

Drug	Starting dose (mg)	Commonest daily dose (mg)	Maintenance range (mg)	Dosage interval[†]
Felbamate	1200	2400	1800–4800	tds
Gabapentin	300–400	2400	1200–4800	tds
Lamotrigine	12.5–50*	200–400	100–800	od–bd
Levetiracetam	1000	2000–3000	1000–4000	bd
Oxcarbazepine	150–600	900–1800	900–2700	bd–tds
Tiagabine	4–10	40	20–60	bd–qds
Topiramate	25–50	200–400	100–1000	bd
Vigabatrin	500–1000	3000	2000–4000	od–bd
Zonisamide	100	400	400–600	od–bd

*12.5 mg with sodium valproate (every other day in the USA). 25 mg as monotherapy
[†]od, once daily; bd, twice daily; tds, three times a day; qds, four times a day

TABLE 5.7

Dosing guidelines for new antiepileptic drugs in children

Drug	Starting dose (mg/kg/day)	Maintenance range (mg/kg/day)	Dose interval[†]
Felbamate	15	30–45	tds–qds
Gabapentin	Not yet recommended for children aged under 12 years		
Lamotrigine	0.2–2*	1.5–15	od–bd
Levetiracetam	Not yet recommended for children aged under 12 years		
Oxcarbazepine	10	10–50	bd–tds
Tiagabine	Not yet recommended for children aged under 12 years		
Topiramate			
UK	25 mg nocte	5–9	bd
USA	0.5–1 (od)	6–9	bd
Vigabatrin	40	50–150	od–bd
Zonisamide	2–4	4–8	bd

*0.2 mg/kg/day when administered with sodium valproate
[†]od, once daily; bd, twice daily; tds, three times a day; qds, four times a day

which is more likely in patients already taking VPA. To date, there is no evidence that LTG is teratogenic.

LTG does not influence the metabolism of lipid-soluble drugs, including other AEDs, warfarin and the oral contraceptive pill. As monotherapy, the half-life approximates 24 hours. When LTG is given to patients already being treated with the enzyme-inducing agents CBZ, PHT or PB, the half-life is about 15 hours. VPA inhibits LTG's glucuronidation, prolonging its half-life to around 60 hours. Withdrawal of enzyme-inducing AEDs causes a rise in the circulating concentrations of LTG, while discontinuing VPA produces a fall. In these circumstances, concentration monitoring may be helpful in guiding LTG dose adjustment. A pharmacodynamic interaction resulting in symptoms of neurotoxicity (headache, dizziness, nausea, diplopia, ataxia) is a common consequence when LTG is introduced in patients established on high-dose CBZ. Patients should be advised to reduce the CBZ dose or stagger the LTG and CBZ doses if they develop neurotoxic symptoms. A pharmacodynamic interaction has also been proposed as the explanation for the marked tremor seen in some patients taking VPA and LTG in combination.

LTG can be administered once daily as monotherapy and with VPA, or twice daily in patients being treated with enzyme-inducing AEDs. A low starting dose with a slow titration schedule should be employed to reduce the risk of rash. This depends on concomitant medication (Table 5.9). Some patients respond to and tolerate LTG doses exceeding 600 mg daily as monotherapy, or above 800 mg daily in combination with an enzyme-inducing AED. An equivalent high dose in VPA-treated patients would be 150–200 mg daily because of the extent of metabolic inhibition. With the above exception, routine concentration monitoring is not required, as no useful relationship has been established between LTG concentrations and its anticonvulsant efficacy or the emergence of side-effects.

TABLE 5.8

Efficacy of new antiepileptic drugs against common seizure types and syndromes

Drug	Partial	Secondary generalized	Tonic–clonic	Absence	Myoclonic	Lennox-Gastaut	Infantile spasms
Felbamate	+	+	?+	?+	?	+	?
Gabapentin	+	+	?+	–	–	?	?
Lamotrigine	+	+	+	+	+	+	?+
Levetiracetam	+	+	+	?+	?+	?	?
Oxcarbazepine	+	+	+	–	–	0	0
Tiagabine	+	+	?	?	?	?	?+
Topiramate	+	+	+	?	+	+	?+
Vigabatrin	+	+	?+	–	–	?	+
Zonisamide	+	+	+	?+	?+	?+	?+

+, proven efficacy; ?+, probable efficacy; 0, ineffective; –, worsens control; ?, unknown

TABLE 5.9

Lamotrigine dosing and titration schedules

Add-on in treated Concomitant antiepileptic drugs

Adults

	Valproate	Others
Weeks 1 and 2	12.5 mg daily (12.5 mg every other day more common in USA)	50 mg daily
Weeks 3 and 4	25 mg daily (12.5 mg daily more common in USA)	50 mg twice daily
Maintenance	50–100 mg* twice daily	100–200 mg* twice daily

Children

	Valproate	Others
Weeks 1 and 2	0.15 mg/kg	0.6 mg/kg
Weeks 3 and 4	0.3 mg/kg	1.2 mg/kg
Increments	0.3 mg/kg	1.2 mg/kg
Maintenance	1–5 mg/kg*	5–15 mg/kg*

Monotherapy

	Adults	Children
Weeks 1 and 2	25 mg daily	0.5 mg/kg
Weeks 3 and 4	25 mg twice daily	1 mg/kg
Maintenance	50–100 mg* twice daily	2–8 mg/kg*

*Higher doses can be tried if seizures persist and the patient is tolerating the drug well

Gabapentin was formed by the addition of a cyclohexyl group to GABA, which allowed it to cross the blood–brain barrier. Despite its structure, GBP does not bind to GABA receptors in the CNS. Its mechanism of action is unknown. GBP is approved as adjunctive therapy for partial seizures with or without secondary generalization in patients 12 years of age and older. It has recently been licensed as monotherapy for the same indications in some countries. It may exacerbate myoclonic jerks and generalized absences.

GBP is not metabolized, and does not induce or inhibit hepatic enzymes. Drug interactions, therefore, are not an issue with this drug. Its half-life is 4–9 hours. Because GBP is eliminated unchanged by the kidneys, patients with renal insufficiency need lower doses and less frequent dosing. A useful serum concentration range has not been established.

Side-effects with GBP are generally mild and transient. Drowsiness, ataxia, dizziness and nystagmus are the most common. Weight gain occurs in up to 5% of patients. At high doses, flatulence, diarrhoea and myoclonic jerks have been reported. No idiosyncratic reactions or effects on bone-marrow or hepatic function have been described. Dosing should be initiated at 300 mg or 400 mg a day and increased by 300 mg or 400 mg increments every 1–3 days to the maximum tolerated dose using a three times daily regimen. The recommended dose range is 1200–2400 mg daily (900–1800 mg daily in the US). However, many patients with refractory epilepsy will need higher amounts (up to 4800 mg daily) for optimal seizure control.

Vigabatrin's antiepileptic effect is mediated by suicidal inhibition of GABA transaminase, the enzyme responsible for the metabolic degradation of GABA (Figure 5.4). It does not interfere with hepatic metabolic enzymes, but produces a small reduction in PHT levels of around 20% by an unknown mechanism. VGB is an effective add-on drug for patients with partial seizures with or without secondary generalization. It can worsen myoclonic jerks and generalized absences. VGB is regarded by many paediatric specialists as the treatment of choice for infantile spasms with more than 50% of children being reported as spasm-free after 1 week of treatment. Children with tuberous sclerosis often have a particularly favourable response. Studies are ongoing to explore its effect on the long-term outcome of this often devastating seizure disorder.

Tiredness, dizziness, headache and weight gain are the most frequent adverse effects with VGB. Some patients report a change in mood, commonly agitation, ill temper, disturbed behaviour or depression. Paranoid and psychotic symptoms can develop, and so patients with a psychiatric history should be treated cautiously with the drug. Hyperkinesia and agitation can occur in children. No idiosyncratic reactions have been reported with VGB. About 25% of patients taking VGB have developed bilateral visual field constriction. This 'tunnel vision' is likely to represent an unusual side-effect of the drug by an unknown mechanism. Accordingly, visual fields should be monitored in patients starting on the drug. There is no evidence that VGB is a human teratogen.

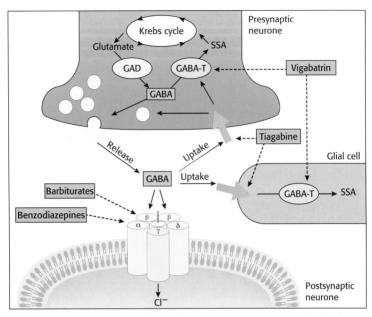

Figure 5.4 Effects of vigabatrin and tiagabine at the GABA$_A$ receptor. Vigabatrin inhibits GABA-T, which degrades GABA, and tiagabine blocks pre-synaptic neuronal and glial uptake of synaptically released GABA. GABA, γ-aminobutyric acid; GABA-T, GABA transaminase; GAD, glutamic acid decarboxylase; SSA, succinic semi-aldehyde. With permission from Leach JP and Brodie MJ. Tiagabine. © *The Lancet* 1998;351:204.

VGB is usually added to existing AED therapy, initially in a dose of 500 mg once or twice daily to allow tolerance to any sedation. If the patient complains of agitation or a thought disorder, the drug should be withdrawn immediately. Further increments of 500 mg or 1000 mg daily will depend on the clinical status of the patient. Seizures in most patients will respond to 2000–3000 mg VGB daily. Few show further improvement at higher doses. Children should be commenced on 40 mg/kg daily, increased according to response up to 80–100 mg/kg daily. Infants with spasms may need as much as 150 mg/kg daily. When being discontinued, VGB should be tapered slowly, as abrupt cessation can produce a marked increase in seizures and precipitate psychosis. Monitoring of VGB concentrations is unnecessary as the drug does not exhibit a useful concentration–effect–toxicity relationship.

Topiramate is a sulphamate-substituted monosaccharide that has a triple pharmacological action involving blockade of sodium channels, attenuation of kainate-induced responses and enhancement of GABA-ergic neurotransmission. It also inhibits carbonic anhydrase, an effect that contributes to its side-effect profile. TPM inhibits the metabolism of PHT in about 10% of patients and accelerates the breakdown of the oestrogenic component of the oral contraceptive pill. PHT and CBZ themselves induce TPM degradation, reducing its concentration by 40% or more. TPM has proven efficacy for partial and tonic–clonic seizures. It seems effective also in the myoclonic epilepsies including some of the more severe syndromes of childhood. A useful effect on generalized absences has yet to be shown. However, it can provide benefit to patients with Lennox-Gastaut syndrome and possibly also infantile spasms.

TPM can produce CNS side-effects including ataxia, poor concentration, confusion, dysphasia, dizziness, fatigue, paraesthesia, somnolence, word-finding difficulties and cognitive slowing. Anorexia and weight loss are common accompaniments of TPM therapy. It increases the risk of nephrolithiasis ten-fold and, therefore, should be avoided in patients with a history of kidney stones and in those taking calcium supplements or high-dose vitamin C. In preclinical studies involving mice, rats and rabbits, TPM was found to be teratogenic at high doses. Its use is, therefore, not advised in pregnancy, unless the benefits of treatment are felt to outweigh the potential risk to the fetus.

Patients respond to TPM in doses ranging from 50–1000 mg daily. It is administered in two divided doses and should be introduced slowly. An initial dose of 25–50 mg daily can be increased by 25–50 mg every 1–2 weeks until a maximally effective and/or tolerated dose is achieved. The optimum amount for most patients with refractory epilepsy appears to be 200–400 mg twice daily. Higher doses (400–800 mg daily) may be required in patients taking PHT or CBZ, with lower amounts (100–200 mg) often being successful in those taking non-inducing AEDs. Some patients respond to doses as low as 50–100 mg daily, particularly if combined with lamotrigine. Concentration monitoring of TPM is not required. However, measurement of PHT levels may be necessary in patients who develop symptoms suggestive of toxicity. Women taking an oral contraceptive should use a formulation containing at least 50 μg ethinyloestradiol. 47

Tiagabine selectively inhibits the neuronal and glial reuptake of GABA and, therefore, enhances GABA-mediated inhibition (see Figure 5.4). It is rapidly and completely absorbed. Food reduces the rate, but not the extent, of absorption. TGB is extensively metabolized by hepatic oxidization via the cytochrome P450 isoenzyme CYP3A. Because TGB does not induce or inhibit liver enzymes, concentrations of CBZ, PHT, theophylline, warfarin and digoxin are unaffected. VPA levels may drop slightly by an unknown mechanism. Its half-life is 5–9 hours, which falls to 2–4 hours when TGB is coadministered with hepatic enzyme-inducing AEDs, such as CBZ and PHT. TGB undergoes linear pharmacokinetics that do not vary significantly in the elderly. Children eliminate TGB slightly faster than adults. Lower doses are required in patients with significant hepatic, but not renal, impairment.

Adverse effects with TGB include dizziness, asthenia (fatigue or muscle weakness), nervousness, tremor, impaired concentration, mental lethargy and depression. Weakness due to transient loss of tone can occur at high doses. The commonest reasons for discontinuation of therapy are confusion, somnolence, ataxia and dizziness. The rates of occurrence for rash and psychosis were similar for TGB-treated patients and those taking placebo in clinical trials. The safety of TGB in pregnancy is unknown, but it is not teratogenic in animals at therapeutic doses.

TGB is licensed throughout the European Union and has been approved for use in the USA as add-on therapy in refractory partial epilepsy. It is available as 5 mg, 10 mg and 15 mg tablets, except in the USA, Canada and Mexico where 2 mg, 4 mg, 12 mg, 16 mg and 20 mg tablets of TGB have been produced. Studies suggest a minimal effective dose of around 20–30 mg/day as add-on in partial epilepsy. The dose range most extensively studied has been 32–56 mg/day, but some patients have demonstrated benefit with up to 80 mg TGB daily. Dosing is likely to be substantially lower when the drug is used as monotherapy. Treatment in adults is started with 4–5 mg once or twice daily, followed by weekly increments of 4–5 mg. A change to three times daily dosing is recommended when 30 mg or more of the drug is prescribed daily. TGB should be taken with food to avoid rapid rises in plasma concentration. Routine plasma level monitoring is not required.

Oxcarbazepine, the 10-keto analogue of CBZ, is licensed in more than 50 countries, including the UK and USA recently. It is functionally a prodrug, being rapidly reduced in the liver to the active metabolite 10,11-dihydro-10-hydroxy-CBZ. Its major effect is to prevent burst firing of neurones by blocking sodium channels, but it also modulates calcium and potassium currents. OXC has no effect on its own metabolism, but it induces a single isoform of cytochrome P450 resulting in accelerated clearance of the hormonal components of the oral contraceptive pill.

OXC has a similar spectrum of efficacy to CBZ against partial and tonic–clonic seizures. It tends to be better tolerated than CBZ with fewer neurotoxic side-effects. Adverse events with OXC most often involve the CNS and include drowsiness, dizziness, headache, diplopia, nausea, vomiting and ataxia. Rash occurs less frequently with OXC than with CBZ. OXC does not appear to produce blood dyscrasias or hepatotoxicity. Hyponatraemia, probably secondary to an antidiuretic hormone-like effect, is as common with OXC as with CBZ, although affected patients are rarely symptomatic. There is no evidence that OXC is a human teratogen, though high doses produce malformations in rodents.

The recommended starting dose for OXC in adults is 150–600 mg daily in two divided doses using the new formulation. The dose can be titrated upwards as clinically indicated to 3000–4000 mg daily. A starting dose of 10 mg/kg daily in children over 3 years can initially be prescribed, increasing gradually to a maintenance amount of about 30 mg/kg daily. Plasma concentrations of the clinically active metabolite of OXC increase linearly with dose. No studies, however, have attempted to relate these with efficacy or toxicity.

Felbamate was the first new AED to be approved in the USA since VPA. It has been shown to be effective as monotherapy and add-on for partial-onset and tonic–clonic seizures in patients 14 years of age and older. It also has important efficacy as adjunctive therapy in the treatment of partial and generalized seizures (including atonic seizures) associated with the Lennox-Gastaut syndrome in children. FBM potentiates GABA activity and blocks voltage-dependent sodium channels as well as the ionic channel at the N-methyl-D-aspartate excitatory amino-acid receptor. FBM is 25% bound to plasma protein and is approximately 50% metabolized by the hepatic cytochrome P450 system. Its half-life ranges between 15 and 24 hours. FBM increases serum concentrations of PHT, VPA and CBZ epoxide. Thus, dose adjustment of concomitant AEDs is usually necessary when FBM is introduced.

Typical side-effects are insomnia, headache, nausea, anorexia, somnolence, vomiting, weight loss and dizziness. Clinical experience with FBM subsequent to its approval by the Food and Drug Administration in the USA showed a significant incidence of aplastic anaemia and hepatotoxicity. As a result, the use of FBM is now largely restricted to patients with Lennox-Gastaut syndrome for whom the benefits of treatment outweigh the risks. Dosing should be initiated slowly and titrated over several weeks to minimize side-effects. Doses of 1800–4800 mg daily in adults and 15–45 mg/kg daily in children are usually necessary for optimal seizure control. Routine monitoring of liver and bone-marrow function is recommended, but will not fully predict the occurrence of potentially fatal toxicity.

Levetiracetam, an enantiomer of the ethyl analogue of piracetam, has an unknown pharmacological action. It is less than 10% protein-bound and the major metabolic pathway is hydrolysis of the acetamide group to the inactive carboxylic derivative. Because its metabolism is independent of the hepatic cytochrome P450 system, there are no pharmacokinetic interactions with other drugs, including oral contraceptives. Steady state is achieved after 2 days of twice-daily dosing. Children aged 6–12 years clear LEV faster than adults. In young adults, the half-life is 7–8 hours compared with 10–11 hours in the healthy elderly, who have age-related diminished renal function. LEV has proven efficacy for treatment-resistant partial seizures. There is suggestive evidence of efficacy in a variety of generalized seizure types, including myoclonic jerks and absences.

In controlled studies, patients with partial seizures responded to LEV 1000–3000 mg daily. Daily doses of up to 4000 mg appear to be well tolerated. Treatment can be initiated at 500 mg twice daily and titrated at 1000 mg increments every 2 weeks as tolerated and needed for seizure control. Because urinary excretion of unchanged drug accounts for approximately 60% of the administered dose, patients with moderate to severe renal impairment may need lower amounts at longer intervals. LEV can produce somnolence, dizziness, headache, anorexia and nervousness. No idiosyncratic reactions with the drug have been reported to date.

Zonisamide is a sulfonamide derivative, which is chemically and structurally unrelated to other AEDs. It blocks voltage-dependent sodium and T-type calcium channels, and actively inhibits the release of excitatory neurotransmitters. It also weakly inhibits carbonic anhydrase activity, which, though probably not a major contributor to ZNS's pharmacological effect, may contribute to its side-effect profile. There is experimental evidence of a possible neuroprotective effect. ZNS binding to protein in serum is approximately 40%, which is unaffected by tightly protein-bound drugs, and it has no effect on hepatic metabolism. It has a high affinity for erythrocytes and this binding is saturable; the relationship between the dose and whole blood ZNS concentration is therefore non-linear at high dosage. The plasma half-life of ZNS ranges from 50 to 68 hours and so steady state is achieved in about 15 days. Children require higher daily doses than adults to achieve comparable serum concentrations because of faster clearance. Patients with renal dysfunction have lower rates of clearance. Enzyme-inducing AEDs, such as PHT, CBZ and PB, decrease the half-life of ZNS by approximately 50%.

ZNS has proven efficacy for treatment-resistant partial seizures. There is evidence suggestive of efficacy for infantile spasms and a variety of generalized seizure types, including tonic–clonic, tonic, atonic and atypical absence seizures. Anecdotal reports suggest that ZNS may have important benefits against seizures in patients with progressive myoclonic epilepsy. With regard to its side-effect profile, ZNS can produce anorexia, dizziness, ataxia, fatigue, somnolence, confusion and poor concentration. Gastrointestinal problems and loss of or decrease in spontaneity have been described. Around 2% of treated patients develop renal stones that may resolve spontaneously.

The recommended initial dose for ZNS is 100 mg daily for adult patients and 2 mg/kg/day for children in two divided dosages. Because steady state is reached slowly, the dose should be increased at 2-week intervals to a target maintenance amount of 400–600 mg/day in adults and 4–8 mg/kg/day in children. Therapeutic drug monitoring with this drug may prove useful.

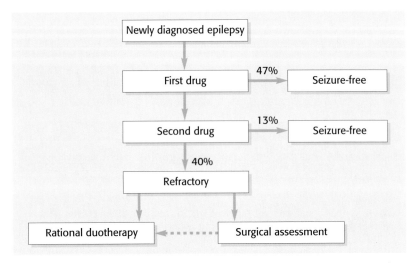

Figure 5.5 Strategies for managing newly diagnosed epilepsy. Data from Kwan and Brodie. *N Engl J Med* 2000;342:314–19.

Choice of treatment

Monotherapy. Seizures in around 60% of patients with newly diagnosed epilepsy will be controlled with the first- or second-choice AED. Most of the remaining patients will need combination therapy (Figure 5.5). In comparison with combination therapy, monotherapy is associated with better compliance and fewer side-effects and is, therefore, also likely to be more cost-effective. For these reasons, monotherapy trials of two AEDs that are first line for the patient's seizure type(s) should be initiated before combinations are tried. Drug choices in adults and children are shown in Tables 5.10 and 5.11. Doses should be slowly titrated to those maximally tolerated. Measuring AED serum concentrations can be helpful in ensuring compliance, in assessing side-effects, and in establishing the therapeutic concentration in a seizure-free patient. Serum concentrations of AEDs that are associated with optimal control or with neurotoxicity vary from patient to patient and may occur below, within or above the so-called 'therapeutic' or 'target' ranges for the drugs, particularly in children and elderly patients. These ranges should be regarded, therefore, purely as a guide to prescribing. Measurement of free serum PHT and VPA concentrations can occasionally be useful when patients have low serum albumin levels or take other tightly protein-bound medications. Women with exacerbation of seizures just prior

TABLE 5.10

Drug choice in newly diagnosed epilepsy in adolescents and adults

Seizure type	First line	Second line
Tonic–clonic	• Sodium valproate • Carbamazepine • Phenytoin	• Lamotrigine* • Oxcarbazepine*
Absence	• Sodium valproate	• Ethosuximide • Lamotrigine*
Myoclonic	• Sodium valproate	• Lamotrigine*
Partial	• Carbamazepine • Phenytoin	• Lamotrigine* • Oxcarbazepine* • Sodium valproate
Unclassifiable	• Sodium valproate	• Lamotrigine*

*Lamotrigine and oxcarbazepine are regarded as first-line drugs in some countries

to their menses should have serum AED concentrations checked in the premenstrual period and compared with mid-cycle concentrations, as they can drop significantly just before and during menstruation.

Rational combinations. Before prescribing combination AED therapy because of lack of efficacy, the clinician should consider why a patient's seizures have not responded to treatment. Possible reasons are listed in Table 5.12. If treatment with two first-line AEDs as monotherapy proves ineffective, achieving complete seizure control with additional monotherapy trials is unlikely. Some patients show useful improvement in seizure frequency or severity with a combination of AEDs particularly using an established with a newer agent. The goal is to maximize efficacy and minimize side-effects. The number of possible two-drug regimens is growing rapidly. Increasing evidence supporting, in particular, the beneficial effects of VPA with LTG is mounting. Many specialists will combine AEDs that have different mechanisms of action for patients with more than one seizure type, and drugs with similar mechanisms when there is a single type of seizure that proves refractory to monotherapy. Some useful examples are listed in Table 5.13. The practical difficulty with combination therapy is

TABLE 5.11

Choice of antiepileptic drugs in children*

Seizure type	First line	Second line	Third line
Tonic–clonic	• Sodium valproate • Carbamazepine	• Lamotrigine* • Oxcarbazepine*	• Phenytoin
Myoclonic	• Sodium valproate	• Lamotrigine*	• Clobazam[†] • Phenobarbital
Tonic	• Sodium valproate	• Lamotrigine*	• Clobazam[†] • Topiramate
Absence	• Sodium valproate	• Lamotrigine* • Ethosuximide	• Clobazam[†]
Partial	• Carbamazepine • Phenytoin	• Sodium valproate • Gabapentin • Oxcarbazepine*	• Lamotrigine • Vigabatrin[†] • Clobazam[†] • Topiramate
Infantile spasms	• Vigabatrin[†] • Corticosteroids	• Sodium valproate • Nitrazepam[†]	• Lamotrigine
Lennox-Gastaut	• Sodium valproate	• Lamotrigine* • Topiramate	• Clobazam[†] • Felbamate

*Lamotrigine and oxcarbazepine are regarded as first-line drugs in some countries
[†]Not approved in the USA

that troublesome or disabling side-effects are common. Consequently, combinations of drugs with different side-effect profiles and those that do not have potential for deleterious drug interactions are advisable. Practical guidelines for prescribing AEDs are summarized in Table 5.14.

When to refer

The primary goal of epilepsy management is to restore the patient's functional capacity to maximal potential. Attaining this goal is often a team effort involving medical and social service professionals and the patient's family, friends and co-workers. The role of the family physician varies according to the clinical setting, his/her experience and the patient's needs. It is important for primary care physicians to be familiar with current diagnostic and therapeutic options.

TABLE 5.12

Some reasons for failure of monotherapy

Wrong diagnosis

- Syncope, cardiac arrhythmia, etc.
- Malingering, pseudoseizures
- Underlying neoplasm

Wrong drug(s)

- Inappropriate for seizure type
- Kinetic/dynamic interactions

Wrong dose

- Too low (ignore target range)
- Side-effects preventing dose increase

Wrong patient

- Poor compliance with medication
- Inappropriate lifestyle (e.g. alcohol or drug abuse)

Initial evaluation of the first seizure can be performed by the family physician, primarily to exclude non-epileptic causes such as syncope and hypoglycaemia. Even experienced family physicians may not feel qualified, however, to assume full responsibility for the diagnosis, planning and follow up of patients with epilepsy. Often, they do not have direct access

TABLE 5.13

Combinations of drugs reported to be useful in refractory epilepsy

Combination	Indication
Sodium valproate and ethosuximide	Generalized absences
Carbamazepine and sodium valproate	Complex partial seizures
Sodium valproate and lamotrigine	Partial/generalized seizures
Vigabatrin and lamotrigine	Partial seizures
Vigabatrin and tiagabine	Partial seizures
Topiramate and lamotrigine	Refractory epilepsy

TABLE 5.14

Ten commandments in the pharmacological treatment of epilepsy

- Choose the correct drug for the seizure type or epilepsy syndrome
- Start at low dosage and increase incrementally
- Titrate slowly to allow tolerance to central nervous system side-effects
- Keep the regimen simple with once- or twice-daily dosing, if possible
- Measure drug concentration when seizures are controlled or if control is not readily obtained (if possible)
- Counsel the patient early regarding the implications of the diagnosis and the prophylactic nature of drug therapy
- Try two reasonable monotherapy options before adding a second drug
- When seizures persist, combine the best tolerated first-line drug with one of the newer agents depending on seizure type and mechanism of action
- Simplify dose schedules and drug regimens as much as possible in patients receiving polypharmacy
- Aim for the best seizure control consistent with the optimal quality of life in patients with refractory epilepsy

to the necessary investigations. If a non-epileptic cause for the symptoms is ruled out, the patient should undergo a consultation by a neurologist or other appropriate specialist to obtain diagnostic studies, determine the likelihood of further seizures, and consider the need for and choice of AED therapy. Dose adjustments can later be undertaken by the family physician. Referral back to the epilepsy specialist should occur if complete seizure control without side-effects is not obtained, when a female patient is planning a pregnancy, or if a seizure-free patient is considering withdrawal of therapy.

Attending to the psychosocial, cognitive, educational and vocational aspects is an important part of caring for people with epilepsy. The family physician and epilepsy specialist should work closely with other medical and social service professionals, and extend their roles beyond that of clinician to patient educator and advocate. Subsequent referral to a comprehensive epilepsy centre for EEG monitoring, investigational drugs or consideration of epilepsy surgery is indicated for compliant patients whose seizures prove refractory to all reasonable attempts at pharmacological manipulation using new and established AEDs singly and in combination.

CHAPTER 6
Special populations

Teenagers

Some types of epilepsy, such as the idiopathic syndromes juvenile myoclonic epilepsy and generalized tonic–clonic seizures upon awakening, are more likely to manifest during the teenage years. Sleep deprivation, photosensitivity and major stresses such as school examinations are common triggers. Partial seizures can also present during teenage years, either *de novo* or as a recurrence of a dormant childhood condition, such as mesial temporal sclerosis. This structural abnormality may be a consequence of one or more prolonged febrile convulsions in infancy or a manifestation of underlying cortical dysplasia. LTG is a good initial choice of treatment for teenagers because it:

- has a wide spectrum of activity
- is particularly well tolerated
- does not interact with the hormonal components of the oral contraceptive pill.

In addition, there is emerging evidence that LTG will prove to be non-teratogenic.

Children who develop epilepsy should be re-evaluated during their teenage years. As they reach puberty, hepatic metabolism slows to a rate approximating that of adults, which may lead to a rise in AED concentrations in the body. AED doses may therefore need to be reduced. However, such a rise is often offset by a teenage growth spurt. If monitoring shows AED levels beginning to fall, this may indicate imperfect compliance, a common occurrence in this age group. The teenage years too are an appropriate time for counselling on contraception, clarifying possible side-effects of AED, and predicting prognosis and eventual drug withdrawal. Driving, social interactions and career advice are other issues that doctors caring for teenagers with epilepsy must address.

Women of childbearing age

The choice of therapy for women during their childbearing years is influenced by the affect of AED treatment on hormones, sexuality and pregnancy. AED treatment reduces fertility rates to one-third of their non-epileptic siblings. Up to 20% of women with epilepsy have abnormal ovarian function, including anovulatory menstrual cycles and polycystic ovaries. These problems may be more common in patients treated with VPA.

Contraception. CBZ, PHT, PB, PRM, TPM, OXC and FBM all induce the metabolism of female sex hormones, which can lead to an altered menstrual cycle and increased turnover of the components of oral contraceptive pills and depot formulations of steroid hormones. The risk of breakthrough pregnancy is not insignificant. Starting with an oral contraceptive formulation containing 50 µg oestrogen, with subsequent adjustment depending on the presence or absence of breakthrough bleeding, can provide secure contraception. Other birth control measures must be taken until the pattern of menstruation has been stable for at least 3 months.

Levonorgestrel implants are contraindicated in women taking enzyme-inducing AEDs as they have an unacceptably high failure rate. This is also likely to be the case with the progesterone-only pill. Medroxyprogesterone injections appear to be effective, though they may need to be given more frequently than is usually recommended. The morning-after contraceptive pill can be used after unprotected intercourse. Issues surrounding pregnancy and lactation are discussed separately in Chapter 7.

Menstruation. Some women find that their seizures exacerbate around menstruation, a phenomenon known as catamenial epilepsy. This is thought to be a consequence of imbalance between the proconvulsant oestrogen and anticonvulant progestogen concentrations. Manipulating the cycle with hormonal preparations is often unsuccessful, however, and may cause unwanted effects such as weight gain and depression. Another option is intermittent CLB just before and shortly after the onset of menstruation.

Reduced bone density. Long-term AED therapy can produce osteomalacia and osteoporosis, which are due in part to induced vitamin D metabolism. However, a reduction in bone density also occurs in women who have only ever received non-inducing AEDs. Vitamin D and calcium supplements should be prescribed if there is evidence of reduced bone density, assuming of course that patients are routinely screened. Bone densitometry should certainly be undertaken in all women sustaining a fracture, whether or not it is seizure-related.

Elderly patients

Old age is the most common time to develop epilepsy. The majority of seizures occurring *de novo* in elderly people are partial in onset with or without secondary generalization. Underlying factors include cerebrovascular disease, intracerebral haemorrhage, dementia and tumour. The aetiology sometimes remains obscure. The diagnosis of epilepsy can be challenging and may have to await a witnessed event. Postictal confusion can be prolonged in the elderly and may contribute to physical injury sustained during a seizure.

AED therapy is the mainstay of treatment, and low doses will help to minimize adverse effects. The patient, and often their spouse and children, must be convinced of the need for lifelong treatment. Choice of drug depends on the side-effect and interaction profiles. A recent double-blind trial supported LTG over CBZ in the elderly. VPA is a suitable alternative, as it is also well tolerated in this population and produces fewer interactions than CBZ or PHT. Complete seizure control can be expected in more than 70% of patients. A subgroup, often with progressive neurodegenerative disease, will continue to have seizures despite all attempts at pharmacological prevention. Sympathetic explanation and assured support will help an elderly person regain his or her self-confidence after epilepsy has been diagnosed and AED treatment established.

Patients with learning disabilities

Epilepsy has the highest prevalence in people with learning disabilities, ranging from 5% in mildly affected individuals to 75% if there is coexistent severe cerebral palsy or postnatal brain injury. Diagnosis relies heavily on an accurate description of events as routine investigations are rarely helpful. Tonic–clonic seizures are common, but many patients also have partial and other generalized seizure types. The clinical picture is often complicated by stereotypies and behavioural disorders. Co-prescribing antipsychotic drugs may further reduce the seizure threshold.

Prior to the first hospital appointment, a great deal of useful information can be obtained from a home assessment by an epilepsy nurse specialist following an agreed protocol. This should include a description of the episodes, an IQ assessment, details of concomitant medication, previous and current AED treatment, circulating AED levels if appropriate, carer's concerns and so on. Home video recordings can help to confirm or refute the epilepsy diagnosis. At the outset, a management plan, including outcome aims, should be formulated with the full involvement of the carers and family. Numbers and doses of AEDs should be rationalized. Attention should be paid not only to seizure frequency and severity, but also to behaviour, mood, appetite, communication, cooperation, alertness and sleep pattern. Broad-spectrum AEDs, such as VPA, LTG and TPM, should be preferred, and barbiturates and benzodiazepines avoided. The end-point need not always be freedom from seizures, but perhaps better control accompanied by improved alertness, mood and cooperation.

CHAPTER 7
Pregnancy

Most pregnant women with treated epilepsy can expect to undergo uneventful pregnancies and deliver healthy babies. During pregnancy, however, metabolic processes change and close attention needs to be given to AED concentrations. Total serum concentrations of some drugs will fall, particularly those of PHT (Figure 7.1) and LTG. Women whose epilepsy is well controlled usually remain seizure-free during pregnancy and delivery. However, those who continue to report seizures pre-conception may suffer a deterioration during pregnancy.

There is an increased incidence of minor and major fetal malformations in the offspring of epileptic women, even if they are untreated. Commonly quoted figures are 2–3% in the general population compared with 3–6% for women with epilepsy. The risk increases disproportionately with the number of AEDs, being approximately 3% for one drug (similar to background), 5% for two, 10% for three, and over 20% in women taking more than three AEDs (Figure 7.2). A syndrome consisting of facial dimorphism, cleft lip and palate, cardiac defects, digital hypoplasia and nail dysplasia has

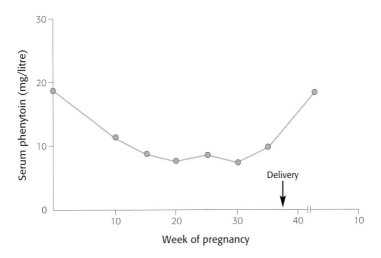

Figure 7.1 Serum phenytoin concentrations during pregnancy and delivery in a woman taking an established dose of 300 mg daily.

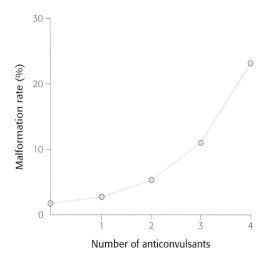

Figure 7.2 Relation of number of antiepileptic drugs taken during the first trimester of pregnancy and the likelihood of fetal malformation. Data from Nakane *et al. Epilepsia* 1980;21:663–80.

been identified. This was initially ascribed to hydantoins including PHT ('fetal-hydantoin syndrome'), but is now known to occur with other AEDs, including CBZ and VPA. There are no clear data indicating differences in safety among PHT, PB or PRM. Current evidence suggests that VPA and CBZ are associated with an increased incidence of neural tube defects of about 1% and 0.5%, respectively. Many of the newer AEDs do not produce malformations when administered to rodents, but it is too early to say whether or not they are human teratogens.

Although it would be ideal for a woman contemplating pregnancy to have AED treatment withdrawn, for many this would result in recurrence or exacerbation of seizures, which can be dangerous for both mother and baby. If the criteria for discontinuation are met, this should be done over a suitable interval before conception (Table 7.1). Drug therapy should be tapered to a minimal effective dose of, if possible, a single AED. In addition, supplemental folic acid should be administered pre-conception in an attempt to prevent neural tube defects. To be effective, folate should be continued for the first 5 weeks of gestation, and the current advice is that it should be taken at least until the end of week 12. Dosage recommendations are 4–5 mg/day folic acid for women with a positive family history of neural tube defects, or who have had a child with such a defect, and 0.4 mg daily in other women planning a pregnancy. It seems sensible, however, to recommend 4–5 mg folate daily for all women receiving treatment with AEDs.

TABLE 7.1

Guidelines for managing epilepsy in pregnancy

- Review the regimen before conception aiming for monotherapy (if possible) with the lowest effective AED dose stressing the importance of planned pregnancy

- Discuss the risks of fetal loss, teratogenesis and development delay with the patient and her partner

- Ensure that potential mothers appreciate that when pregnancy is confirmed, the time for teratogenesis is over and any damage will already have been done

- Discuss available antenatal screening and the need for frequent AED measurements during pregnancy and for at least 8 weeks after delivery

- Prescribe pre-conceptual folic acid (4–5 mg daily for all women with epilepsy) and continue throughout pregnancy

- Point out the risk of haemorrhage disorder in the newborn and the need for oral vitamin K during the last few weeks of pregnancy in women taking enzyme-inducing AEDs

- Discuss the chance of the baby developing epilepsy. Children born to mothers (but not fathers) with epilepsy have a three-fold increased risk of later seizures

- Advise the patient about the need for strict AED compliance and adequate sleep throughout pregnancy

- Document each of the above in the patient's medical record

Enzyme-inducing AEDs (CBZ, PHT, PB and PRM) can cause transient and reversible deficiency in vitamin K-dependent clotting factors in the neonate. Following a traumatic birth, there is an increased risk of intracerebral haemorrhage. Accordingly, babies at risk should receive intramuscular vitamin K_1 immediately after birth, and mothers should take 10 mg vitamin K_1 daily by mouth for the last few weeks of pregnancy.

Pregnancy registry

In the USA. Women with epilepsy who become pregnant should be enrolled in a pregnancy registry. The Antiepileptic Drug Pregnancy Register in the USA was established in 1996 to determine the risk of major malformations from AEDs. Patients should call the toll-free number 001 888 233 2334. Physicians cannot enrol patients; the woman herself must call as part of the informed consent process. There are three brief interviews, lasting 15 minutes initially, 5 minutes at 7 months' gestation and 5 minutes 2–4 weeks postnatally.

In Europe, a similar project is being coordinated. This register requires input from the attending clinician and not the patient. EURAP (European Registry of Antiepileptic Drugs and Pregnancy) is a consortium of independent research groups that have agreed a common protocol for a prospective assessment of pregnancy outcome. All physicians who care for women taking AEDs during pregnancy are invited to contribute. The contact address is dbattino@istituto-besta.it.

CHAPTER 8
Anticonvulsant withdrawal

A successful outcome for a patient with treated epilepsy can be regarded as freedom from seizures without side-effects. Such individuals are more likely to lead rewarding lives, with optimal intellectual and emotional development, and positive educational and vocational achievements than patients with uncontrolled seizures. In short, they will have a better chance of fulfilling their potential. Many can have their medication eventually withdrawn and remain in remission. Patients who are 'doing well' may want to stop treatment for a variety of reasons, including the awareness of side-effects or the subjective perception of subtle deterioration in cognitive function. In addition, some patients do not equate taking medication with normal health. Finally, the patient may want to start a family and may be concerned about the possible negative effects of AEDs on reproductive function and the spectre of teratogenesis.

Several studies have shown that, after a long period of perfect seizure control, medication can be stopped without seizure recurrence (at least over the following several years) in around 60% of patients. There are no data to indicate an optimum length for the seizure-free period. In children, 2 years is reasonable, while in adults a flexible 5 years is more prudent. Seizure type or epilepsy syndrome is not absolutely predictive of recurrence. However, a few specific childhood syndromes, such as benign epilepsy of childhood with rolandic spikes and benign familial neonatal convulsions, tend to do well after drug withdrawal, whereas JME conveys a high probability of relapse. Some forms of idiopathic generalized seizures, either absence or tonic–clonic, are less likely to recur after control is achieved. However, even complex partial seizures can disappear after a long period of freedom from seizures.

Patients with the highest probability of remaining seizure-free include those with relatively few seizures before and after starting AED therapy, those taking a single AED, those seizure-free for many years, and those with a normal neurological examination and no structural lesion on brain imaging. The EEG is not greatly helpful in predicting seizure recurrence, but a normal investigation is reassuring. There are no standard protocols defining optimal regimens for tapering medication. Most specialists advise slow reduction by increments over at least 6 months. If the patient is taking two AEDs, one drug should be slowly withdrawn before the second is tapered. More than 90% of recurrences will occur during the year following withdrawal, and many will present during the tapering period or shortly after.

CHAPTER 9
Status epilepticus

Status epilepticus (SE) is a life-threatening medical emergency defined as frequent and/or prolonged epileptic seizures. Pragmatically, the disorder is diagnosed when patients have continuous or repeated seizure activity without regaining consciousness. Convulsive SE may result from a variety of causes (Table 9.1). The mortality and morbidity reflect the underlying problem and the physiological effects of convulsions, including hypertension, tachycardia, cardiac arrhythmias and hyperthermia; hence the mortality is as high as 10%, rising to 50% in elderly patients. Treatment

TABLE 9.1

Causes of tonic–clonic status epilepticus

Background of epilepsy

- Poor compliance with medication
- Recent change in treatment
- Barbiturate or benzodiazepine withdrawal
- Alcohol or drug abuse
- Pseudostatus epilepticus

Presenting *de novo*

- Recent stroke
- Meningo-encephalitis
- Acute head injury
- Cerebral neoplasm
- Demyelinating disorder
- Metabolic disorders (e.g. renal failure, hypoglycaemia, hypercalcaemia)
- Drug overdose (e.g. tricyclic antidepressants, phenothiazines, theophylline, isoniazid, cocaine)
- Inflammatory arteritides (e.g. systemic lupus erythematosus)

TABLE 9.2

Treatment of convulsive status epilepticus (SE)

1. After two recurrent convulsive seizures without recovery of consciousness in between, the patient should be considered in SE. The same urgency is appropriate when the patient convulses continuously for more than 5 minutes.

2. Establish airway, and ensure adequate respiration, blood pressure and cardiac rhythm. Set up an intravenous line with saline. Administer thiamine and glucose. Give antibiotics when infection is a possibility. Draw blood for metabolic studies, AED levels and toxic screens.

3. Use a long-acting AED. Phenytoin, the most frequently used maintenance medication, can be given in saline at 50 mg/minute, with attention to the cardiogram and blood pressure, to a dose of 18–20 mg/kg or as fosphenytoin in any intravenous fluid up to 150 mg/minute. Alternatively, intravenous phenobarbital may be given at doses of 10–20 mg/kg, up to 100 mg/minute, with attention to blood pressure and respiration.

4. Administer a rapidly acting benzodiazepine (e.g. titrate lorazepam at 2 mg/minute up to 10 mg if SE has lasted 30 minutes and if convulsions occur during phenytoin or phenobarbital infusion). This can be repeated if necessary.

5. Other possible alternatives depending on availability and experience include chlormethiazole, paraldehyde, lignocaine, propofol and midazolam.

6. If SE continues, and after intubation, use pentobarbital 5 mg/kg with the goal of eliminating epileptiform activity on the EEG. Maintenance doses are 1–5 mg/kg/hour as necessary. Consider discontinuing pentobarbital after 24–48 hours, assuming clinical and electrographic seizures have ceased and that one or two longer acting AEDs are at high concentrations.

7. Watch for potential complications of SE, including hypothermia, acidosis, hypotension, rhabdomyolysis, renal failure, infection and cerebral oedema.

8. Continue to search for and treat any underlying cause.

should be initiated immediately (Table 9.2). Delay worsens the prognosis and decreases the likelihood of stopping seizures without having to resort to general anaesthesia. The importance of a coordinated effort involving ambulance technicians, emergency medicine specialists, medical intensivists, and neurological consultants in the treatment of convulsive SE cannot be overemphasized.

Seizure clusters

Some patients experience clusters of seizures (also called acute repetitive seizures), lasting from minutes to hours, that may not be defined by their physicians as SE, yet require therapeutic intervention. Oral therapy, for example with a benzodiazepine, may be problematic and intravenous access is usually unavailable or difficult. Rectal diazepam administered by parents or other caregivers may be effective in this situation. Rectal diazepam is absorbed more rapidly than rectal lorazepam or oral diazepam because of its high lipid solubility. A gel-containing, prefilled, unit-dose rectal delivery system is commercially available. The doses used in clinical studies (0.5 mg/kg for children aged 2–5 years, 0.3 mg/kg for those aged 6–11 years, 0.2 mg/kg for those over 12 years of age) were effective and well tolerated, and did not produce respiratory depression. The most common side-effect was somnolence.

Parents and caregivers must be adequately trained by knowledgeable healthcare professionals to be able to recognize seizure clusters, administer rectal diazepam, monitor the patient for potentially dangerous respiratory depression, and summon emergency medical help when necessary. Excessive usage of rectal diazepam can result in rebound seizures.

CHAPTER 10

Vagus nerve stimulation

The introduction of vagus nerve stimulation (VNS) has provided a new, non-pharmacological approach to epilepsy treatment. Over 7500 patients have been implanted with the NeuroCybernetic Prosthesis® System worldwide with a total cumulative exposure of over 8000 patient years. VNS is approved in the USA, Canada and the 16 European Union countries for use as adjunctive therapy for adults and adolescents over 12 years of age whose partial-onset seizures are refractory to antiepileptic medication. Some patients with generalized seizures will also respond to VNS. The system (Figure 10.1) consists of:

- a programmable signal generator that is implanted in the patient's left upper chest
- a bipolar lead that connects the generator to the left vagus nerve in the neck
- a programming wand that uses radio-frequency signals to communicate non-invasively with the generator
- a hand-held magnet used by the patient or carer to turn the stimulator on or off.

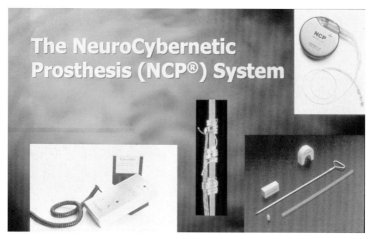

Figure 10.1 A vagus nerve stimulation system. Reproduced with permission from Cyberonics, Inc.

A number of severely affected patients have had clinically significant seizure reductions of over 50% with a few being made seizure-free. There is no indication of tolerance to the therapeutic effect induced by VNS.

The mechanism of action of VNS is unknown. It has no effect on hepatic metabolic processes, serum concentrations of AEDs or laboratory values. VNS does not alter deleteriously vagally mediated physiological processes as measured by Holter monitoring, pulmonary function tests and serum gastrin levels. The implantation procedure lasts approximately 1 hour and is typically carried out under general anaesthesia to minimize the possibility that a seizure will interfere with the surgery. Side-effects are transient and include incisional pain, coughing, voice alteration, chest discomfort and nausea. Adverse effects related to stimulation are usually mild, and almost always resolve with adjustment in the settings. These include hoarseness, throat pain, coughing, dyspnoea and paraesthesia. There have been no reported cognitive, sedative, visual, affective, behavioural or coordination side-effects; hence, conspicuously absent with VNS therapy are the typical CNS problems associated with AEDs.

Within the first 2 postoperative weeks, increasing the output current is initiated by the physician and adjusted to patient tolerance. A typical regimen consists of a 30 Hz signal frequency with a 500-microsecond pulse width for 30 seconds of 'on time' and 5 minutes 'off time'. Once programmed, the generator will deliver intermittent stimulation at the desired settings until any additional instructions are received or until the battery life is expended, which typically occurs after 8–10 years of operation with the latest model. In addition, the patient or a companion may activate the generator by placing the magnet over it for several seconds; in some patients, this may interrupt a seizure or reduce its severity if undertaken at the onset.

CHAPTER 11

Epilepsy surgery

Epilepsy surgery should be considered for patients with medically refractory seizures, particularly when they interfere significantly with their lifestyle. In addition to results of diagnostic tests, the patient's perception of epilepsy severity despite optimal pharmacotherapy and his or her expectations for the future are key determinants in the decision to operate. Indications for commonly undertaken procedures are listed in Table 11.1. The standard approach is intraoperative electrocorticography (Figure 11.1), immediately followed by a cortical excision (lobectomy; see Figures 11.2 and 11.3). The success rate is high when patients are screened carefully; the best results are obtained when the epileptogenic region is localized to the anterior temporal lobe and the MRI is consistent with mesial temporal sclerosis. Most centres report that 70–80% of patients undergoing temporal lobectomy have a marked reduction in seizures, whereas frontal lobectomy produces significant improvement in only 30–40%. At centres in which epilepsy surgery is frequently performed, the incidence of severe complications is generally between 1 and 2%.

There is no universally agreed approach to identifying potential surgical candidates. The definition of what constitutes an adequate trial of

TABLE 11.1

Types of epilepsy surgery and their indications

Procedure	Indication
Focal resection	Partial-onset seizures arising from resectable cortex
Corpus callosotomy	Tonic, atonic or tonic–clonic seizures with falling and injury, large non-resectable lesions, or secondary bilateral synchrony
Hemispherectomy	Rasmussen's syndrome or other unilateral hemisphere pathology in association with functionally impaired contralateral hand
Subpial transections	Partial-onset seizures arising from unresectable cortex

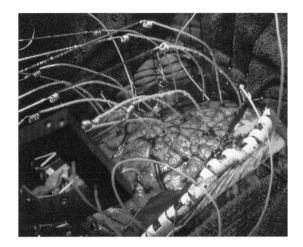

Figure 11.1 EEG electrodes applied to the cortical surface intraoperatively prior to epilepsy surgery.

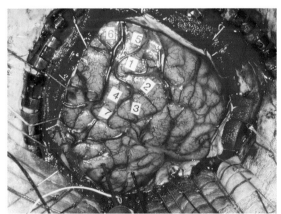

Figure 11.2 A patient prepared for surgery; the area to be resected is clearly marked.

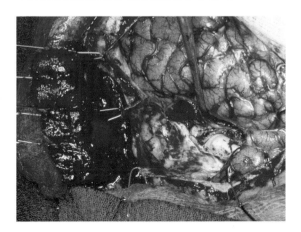

Figure 11.3 Patient in Figure 11.2 immediately after left anterior temporal lobectomy.

medication before surgery varies considerably. However, recent evidence suggests that patients with newly diagnosed partial seizures have a high risk of subsequent refractories if their seizures fail to control on the first two AEDs taken. Patients with operable structural abnormalities should be investigated for surgery early because these lesions tend to cause intractable seizures and surgical success rates are high. Evaluation involves a thorough review of the patient's seizure history and AED trials; sophisticated EEG monitoring to localize the onset of a number of the patient's typical seizures; MRI scanning and, when necessary, functional imaging to delineate a focal structural and/or functional lesion; and neuropsychological testing to identify any cognitive deficits with cerebral localizing significance. Lobar excision may be carried out with a high probability of improvement when:

- EEG monitoring shows that seizure onset is consistently and repeatedly from the same portion of one frontal or temporal lobe
- other investigations are consistent with this localization
- the identified lobe can be removed safely without permanent cognitive, sensory or motor deficit.

If scalp EEG data do not clearly identify the seizure focus, or if the neuroimaging and/or neuropsychological testing results are inconsistent with the ictal results, 'invasive' electrodes may be inserted into the brain for further seizure recording. When monitoring shows that seizures arise from different sides of the brain on separate occasions, or are consistent with generalized seizures, lobectomy is not likely to be of help. Patients with severe generalized seizures, particularly atonic seizures with many falls and subsequent damage, may be candidates for sectioning of the corpus callosum or, on rare occasions, hemispherectomy.

CHAPTER 12

Future trends

With the recent introduction of a range of new AEDs with differing, sometimes single and often multiple, mechanisms of action, there is an imperative to replace the largely empirical approach to the pharmacological management of epilepsy with a more science-based rationale governing drug choice for individual patients. Linked to this must be a better understanding of how seizures are generated and propagated to provide seizure and syndrome classifications that have a neurophysiological and neuropharmacological basis rather than an observational one. These developments will underpin a patient-centred, mechanistic approach to the management of epilepsy. Combining drugs with complementary mechanisms of action will undoubtedly improve the currently unsatisfactory prognosis in refractory epilepsy. This strategy has substantial potential, in particular, to revitalize the management of the malignant encephalopathic syndromes of early childhood, such as Lennox-Gastaut syndrome and infantile spasms.

Current therapy aims to prevent seizures; future treatments may influence the natural history of the epileptic process. The genetics underlying a range of epilepsies are beginning to yield their secrets. This will contribute substantially to the refinement of the seizure and syndrome classifications, and encourage AED development based on pharmacogenomics. The development of 'gene therapy' for the progressive myoclonic epilepsies and other severe seizure syndromes is a long-term goal consequent upon a better understanding of the basis of these disorders.

Appreciation is growing that surgery is the treatment of choice for many patients with lesional epilepsy. This must be performed early before the deleterious effect of repeated seizures produces irreversible neuronal changes, cognitive impairment and psychosocial dysfunction. Surgery is now cost-effective compared with lifelong treatment with one or more of the newer AEDs. The continuing advances in brain imaging are identifying patients suitable for a surgical approach earlier and are also helping to delineate more precisely the target area to be resected. Epilepsy surgery programmes have become an essential component of patient care.

Advances in the understanding, investigation and treatment of epilepsy are continuing apace. There is now substantial potential to ameliorate this distressing disorder in many more patients than ever before. Most people with epilepsy can expect to have their seizures completely controlled without debilitating side-effects. There is an increasingly wide range of medical and surgical strategies to optimize treatment for others with more severe seizure disorders. We have the tools to improve their quality of life. We must learn to use them and the many others that will surely follow during this new millennium.

Key references

EPIDEMIOLOGY

Hauser WA, Annegers JF, Kurland LT. Prevalence of epilepsy in Rochester, Minnesota: 1940–1980. *Epilepsia* 1991;32:429–45.

Hauser WA, Annegers JF, Kurland LT. Incidence of epilepsy and unprovoked seizures in Rochester, Minnesota: 1935–1984. *Epilepsia* 1993;34:453–68.

Kwan P, Brodie MJ. Early identification of refractory epilepsy. *N Engl J Med* 2000;342:314–19.

Leestma JE, Walczak T, Hughes DR *et al.* A prospective study on sudden unexpected death in epilepsy. *Ann Neurol* 1989;26:195–203.

Sander JWAS, Shorvon SD. Epidemiology of the epilepsies. *J Neurol Neurosurg Psychiatry* 1996;6:433–43.

Tallis R, Hall G, Craig I, Dean A. How common are epileptic seizures in old age? *Age Ageing* 1991;20:442–8.

Watts AE. The natural history of untreated epilepsy in a rural community in Africa. *Epilepsia* 1992;33:464–8.

SEIZURES/SYNDROMES

Annegars JF, Hauser WA, Shirts SB *et al.* Factors prognostic of unprovoked seizures after febrile convulsions. *N Engl J Med* 1987;316:493–8.

Commission on Classification and Terminology of the International League Against Epilepsy. Proposal for revised clinical classification of epileptic seizures. *Epilepsia* 1981;22:489–501.

Commission on Classification and Terminology of the International League Against Epilepsy. Proposal for revised clinical classification of epileptic syndromes. *Epilepsia* 1989;30:389–99.

Schachter SC. Update in the treatment of epilepsy. *Comp Ther* 1995;21:473–9.

Schachter SC. Iatrogenic seizures. *Neurol Clin* 1998;16:157–70.

Scheuer ML, Pedley TA. The evaluation and treatment of seizures. *N Engl J Med* 1990;323:1468–73.

GENETICS

Mody I. Ion channels in epilepsy. *Int Rev Neurobiol* 1998;42:199–226.

Prasad AN, Prasad C, Stafstrom CE. Recent advances in the genetics of epilepsy: insights from human and animal studies. *Epilepsia* 1999;40:1329–52.

Scheffer IE, Bhatia KP, Lopes-Cenes I *et al.* Autosomal dominant nocturnal frontal lobe epilepsy. A distinctive clinical disorder. *Brain* 1995;118:61–73.

Scheffer IE, Berkovic SF. Generalised epilepsy with febrile seizures plus. A genetic disorder with heterogeneous clinical phenotypes. *Brain* 1997;120: 479–90.

Singh NA, Charlier C, Stauffer D *et al.* A novel potassium channel gene, KCNQ2, is mutated in an inherited epilepsy of newborns. *Nat Genet* 1998;18:25–9.

Wallace RH, Wang DW, Sing R *et al.*
Febrile seizures and generalised epilepsy
associated with a mutation in the Na$^+$
channel β1 submit gene SCNIB. *Nat
Genet* 1998;19:366–70.

DIAGNOSTIC TECHNIQUES

Binnie CD, Stefan H. Modern
electrophysiology: its role in epilepsy
management. *Clin Neurophysiol*
1999;110:1671–97.

Duncan JS. Imaging epilepsy. *Brain*
1997;120:339–77.

PHARMACOLOGICAL TREATMENT

Brodie MJ, Dichter MA. Antiepileptic
drugs. *N Engl J Med* 1996;334:168–75.

Brodie MJ, Dichter MA. Established
antiepileptic drugs. *Seizure* 1997;
6:159–74.

Brodie MJ, French JA. Management of
epilepsy in adolescents and adults. *Lancet*
2000;356:323–9.

Dichter MA, Brodie MJ. New
antiepileptic drugs. *N Engl J Med*
1996;334:1583–90.

First Seizure Trial Group. Randomised
clinical trial on the efficacy of antiepileptic
drugs in reducing the relapse after a first
unprovoked tonic–clonic seizure.
Neurology 1993;43:478–83.

Marson AG, Kadir ZA, Hutton JL,
Chadwick DW. The new antiepileptic
drugs: a systematic review of their efficacy
and tolerability. *Epilepsia* 1997;38:
859–80.

Mattson RH. Selection of drugs for the
treatment of epilepsy. *Semin Neurol*
1990;10:406–13.

Pellock JM. Managing pediatric epilepsy
syndromes with new antiepileptic drugs.
Pediatrics 1999;104:1106–16.

Perucca E. The new generation of
antiepileptic drugs: advantages and
disadvantages. *Br J Clin Pharmacol*
1996;42:531–43.

Richens A. Rational polypharmacy.
Seizure 1995;4:211–14.

Schachter SC, Yerby MS. The role
of the primary care physician in the
management of epilepsy: guidelines
and tools for patient care. *Postgrad
Med* 1997;101:133–53.

Scheyer RH, Cramer JA.
Pharmacokinetics of antiepileptic drugs.
Semin Neurol 1990;10:313–421.

Schmidt D, Gram L. Monotherapy versus
polytherapy in epilepsy. A reappraisal.
CNS Drugs 1995;3:194–208.

Wilson EA, Brodie MJ. New antiepileptic
drugs. In: Brodie MJ, Treiman DM, eds.
*Modern Management of Epilepsy.
Baillière's Clinical Neurology.* London:
Baillière-Tindall, 1996:723–47.

SPECIAL POPULATIONS

Brodie MJ, Overstall PW, Giorgi L and the
UK Lamotrigine Elderly Study Group.
Multicentre, double-blind, randomised
comparison between lamotrigine and
carbamazepine in elderly patients with
newly diagnosed epilepsy. *Epilepsy Res*
1999;37:81–7.

Crawford P, Appleton R, Betts T *et al.* and
the Women with Epilepsy Guidelines
Development Group. Best practice
guidelines for the management of women
with epilepsy. *Seizure* 1999;8:201–17.

Feely M, Gibson J. Intermittent clobazam for catamenial epilepsy: tolerance avoided. *J Neurol Neurosurg Psychiatry* 1984;27:1279–82.

Hannah JA, Brodie MJ. Epilepsy and learning disabilities – a challenge for the next millennium. *Seizure* 1998;7:3–13.

Stephen LJ, Brodie MJ. Epilepsy in elderly people. *Lancet* 2000;355:1441–6.

Stephen LJ, McLellan AR, Harrison JH *et al*. Bone density and antiepileptic drugs: a case-controlled study. *Seizure* 1999;8: 339–42.

Zahn CA, Morrell MJ, Collins SD *et al*. Management issues for women with epilepsy: a review of the literature. *Neurology* 1998;51:949–56.

PREGNANCY

Brodie MJ. Management of epilepsy during pregnancy and lactation. *Lancet* 1990;336:426–7.

Delgado-Escueta AV, Janz D. Consensus guidelines: pre-conception counselling, management, and care of the pregnant woman with epilepsy. *Neurology* 1992;42:149–60.

Kanner AM, Palac S. Depression in epilepsy: a common but often unrecognized comorbid malady. *Epilepsy Behav* 2000;1:37–51.

Nakane Y, Okuma T, Takahashi R *et al*. Multi-institutional study on the teratogenicity and fetal toxicity of antiepileptic drugs: a report of a collaborative study group in Japan. *Epilepsia* 1980;21:663–80.

Schachter SC. Neuroendocrine aspects of epilepsy. *Neurol Clin* 1994;12:31–40.

Yerby MJ. Contraception, pregnancy and lactation in women with epilepsy. In: Brodie MJ, Treiman DM, eds. *Modern Management of Epilepsy. Baillière's Clinical Neurology*. London: Baillière-Tindall, 1996:887–908.

DRUG WITHDRAWAL

Medical Research Council Antiepileptic Drug Research Group. Randomised study of antiepileptic drug withdrawal in patients in remission. *Lancet* 1991;337: 1175–80.

Shinnar S, Berg AT. Withdrawal of antiepileptic drugs. *Curr Opin Neurol* 1995;8:103–6.

Tennison M, Greenwood R, Lewis D, Thorn M. Rate of taper of antiepileptic drugs and the risk of seizure recurrence in children. *N Engl J Med* 1994;330: 1407–10.

STATUS EPILEPTICUS

Brodtkorb E, Aamo T, Henriksen O, Lossius R. Rectal diazepam: pitfalls of excessive use in refractory epilepsy. *Epilepsy Res* 1999;35:123–33.

Cereghino JJ, Mitchell WG, Murphy J *et al*. Treating repetitive seizures with a rectal diazepam formulation: a randomized study. The North American Diastat Study Group. *Neurology* 1998;51:1274–82.

Dreifuss FE, Rosman NP, Cloyd JC *et al*. A comparison of rectal diazepam gel and placebo for acute repetitive seizures. *N Engl J Med* 1998;338:1869–75.

Mitchell WG. Status epilepticus and acute repetitive seizures in children, adolescents, and young adults: etiology, outcome, and treatment. *Epilepsia* 1996;37(Suppl 1): S74–80.

Shorvon S. Tonic–clonic status epilepticus. *J Neurol Neurosurg Psychiatry* 1993; 56:125–34.

Working group on status epilepticus. Treatment of convulsive status epilepticus. *JAMA* 1993;270:854–9.

VAGUS NERVE STIMULATION

Ben-Menachem E. Vagus nerve stimulation. In: Brodie MJ, Treiman DM, eds. *Modern Management of Epilepsy. Baillière's Clinical Neurology*. London: Baillière-Tindall, 1996:841–8.

Schachter SC. Vagus nerve stimulation. *Epilepsia* 1998;39:677–86.

Uthman BM, Wilder BJ, Penry JK *et al.* Treatment of epilepsy by stimulation of the vagus nerve. *Neurology* 1993;43:1338–45.

EPILEPSY SURGERY

Lesser RP, Fisher RS, Kaplan R. The evaluation of patients with intractable complex partial seizures. *Electroencephalogr Clin Neurophysiol* 1989;73:381–8.

Polkey CE. Surgical treatment of epilepsy. *Lancet* 1990;336:553–5.

Sperling MR, O'Connor MJ, Saykin AJ *et al.* Temporal lobectomy for refractory epilepsy. *JAMA* 1996;276:470–5.

Wyllie E. Corpus callosotomy for intractable generalised epilepsy. *J Pediatr* 1988;113:255–61.

Index

Other titles available in the *Fast Facts* series

To order, please contact:

Health Press Limited
Elizabeth House, Queen Street,
Abingdon, Oxford OX14 3JR, UK
Tel: +44 (0)1235 523233
Fax: +44 (0)1235 523238
Email: post@healthpress.co.uk

Or visit our website:
www.healthpress.co.uk

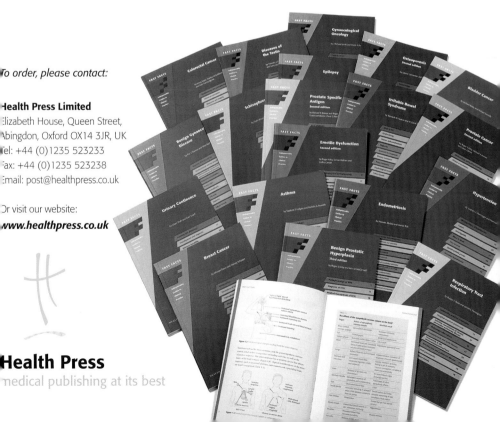

Health Press
medical publishing at its best